HIIT
YOUR LIMIT

HIIT
YOUR LIMIT

HIGH-INTENSITY INTERVAL TRAINING FOR FAT LOSS, CARDIO, AND FULL BODY HEALTH

DR. LEN KRAVITZ

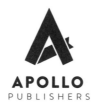

APOLLO
PUBLISHERS

CONTENTS

INTRODUCING A FABULOUS KEY TO HEALTH—

Exercise!

IF THERE EXISTS AN EXQUISITE BLUEPRINT TO ATTAINING HEALTH, WELLNESS, AND LON-gevity, it is a program of regular exercise. No matter who you are or where you are in your life, this blueprint is yours to cherish and embrace daily. The mental and physical benefits of exercise cannot be understated; the pursuit of optimal fitness triggers the development of cardiorespiratory endurance, muscular strength, flexibility, healthy eating patterns, and positive behaviors that spur you to function and perform at your best. Consistent exercise helps bring about a harmonic balance to you as a person and helps you build resilience to the challenges you face in your journey through life. Your level of fitness will determine the quality of your life.

You are in control of how you feel and live. Yes, this is your responsibility. But great news! At any point in your life, you can make lifestyle decisions that noticeably impact your well-being. You are the one who can take the first step to improve your health and promote your wellness through exercise. Thankfully, you do not need megadoses of exercise to realize its many life-changing health benefits. The American College of Sports Medicine (ACSM), the largest sports medicine and exercise science organization in the world, recommends that adults get 150 minutes of moderate (i.e., somewhat hard) exercise per week. That's less time than even a short Netflix binge! Plus, as you will see in this book, you can accumulate your minutes with multiple shorter sessions of at least 10 minutes. The high-intensity interval training (HIIT) programs presented in this book represent some of the most exciting new advances in exercise training. All of the information presented in this book is based on the most contemporary scientific evidence, because I want you to have the best information possible at your fingertips.

Please note that the HIIT workouts in this book are genuine cardiovascular workouts, all adapted from scientific studies. We will discuss some remarkable benefits from HIIT training, including health benefits, fat loss, and disease prevention. However, the word "high-intensity" is a buzzword in the fitness industry for any workout that is very challenging. In fact, if you search "HIIT workouts" on the internet, you may be surprised to see how many different types are shown. Please avoid confusing true cardiovascular HIIT workouts with the many other high-intensity workouts popular today, such as boot camp and body blast.

One of my favorite teaching principles when working with health, fitness, and weight management students and professionals is "Inch by inch, it's a cinch." This is my personal exercise slogan and a philosophy I want to share with you. I established the philosophy as I launched my career in fitness.

Right after I completed my master's degree in physical education at San Jose State University, I landed a fabulous job as fitness director of a new athletic club in Los Gatos, California. Over the next eight years I taught thousands of fitness classes and trained a great many wonderful men, women, boys, and girls. My passion for fitness grew so much that I became well-known in the San Francisco Bay Area for my creative ways of teaching exercise and how much my students enjoyed my classes. It wasn't long before I was invited to fitness conferences around the United States to share my ideas about group fitness exercise classes with other certified fitness professionals. For clarity, the term "group fitness" includes all forms of fitness performed in a group setting and led by a qualified instructor. My circle soon expanded to fitness conferences in Canada, Mexico, Japan, Australia, Brazil, Taiwan, and Europe.

I then laser focused my energy and academic interests to attain my PhD at the University of New Mexico, where I am now an associate professor in the Department of Health, Exercise, and Sports Sciences. My areas of study were health promotion and exercise science.

During my studies a new ambition took hold: improving the education of fitness professionals around the world. Once I realized how meaningful my graduate education was to me, I wanted to pass along my knowledge to others, so I began writing fitness-related articles for industry-leading fitness journals, with a zeal to educate fitness pros throughout the world. The research studies I conducted were focused on solving many of the questions facing fitness professionals. My presentations at conferences also evolved, and I started presenting research-oriented lectures, which remain my focus today.

And here I am today, sharing my story with you. I feel so fortunate that my passion for fitness education has been rewarded in unexpected ways. I currently have over three hundred peer-review articles, I've been invited to present at over one thousand fitness and science conferences throughout the world, and I have been awarded every major honor in the fitness industry, including induction into the National Fitness Hall of Fame. And through it all, with my first students, current students, and all the fitness professionals I have had the pleasure to teach, my mantra has remained "Inch by inch, it's a cinch."

This step-by-step philosophy has proven to be the most successful approach to goal attainment I have ever utilized. I will repeat it multiple times through this book, because it applies to so many aspects of your health, fitness, and weight management—so get ready. I invite you to adopt this slogan for your fitness journey. As catchy as it is, it embodies a proven scientific methodology to weight management called the "small steps" approach, which we will discuss thoroughly in the book. From my professional experiences working with people of all ages and abilities, this process of small steps universally leads to gratifying, successful outcomes that you can sustain. With a modest investment of your time, you can follow the concepts, weight management strategies, and exercise programs in this book and create your ideal fitness plan. All of which is to say, your ultimate power lies with the lifestyle choices you make every day. You can do it!

Before we dive in, I'd like to give you a quick tour of this book. In Section 1: Exercise, HIIT, and You, I cover essential information for launching your journey into fitness, including chapters on the health benefits of exercise; an introduction to HIIT training; the health benefits of HIIT workouts; how to power your HIIT workouts; and how to succeed in exercise and my START MOVING NOW program.

In Section 2: Optimal Weight (Fat) Loss Strategies That Work!, I provide an inspiring and all-inclusive section on weight management. I also cover an important array of hot-button issues related to weight management, energy balance, low-carbohydrate versus low-fat diets, dieting and longevity, and stress and obesity. In the same section I present fascinating weight management information from a landmark study on over ten thousand of the biggest real-life weight loss losers, and I summarize the common strategies they stick to in their daily life. I also answer fifty common questions on health, nutrition, and weight management. These questions come from actual fitness fans, just like you.

Section 3: Let's HIIT the Workouts! presents the magnificent HIIT workouts in all their sweaty, life-improving glory, and includes a guide on how to train properly. All of these workouts are drawn from research studies, and I have adapted them specifically for *all* fitness levels. Yes, there is a way to adapt HIIT workouts for all fitness levels by using a perceived exertion model to gauge your exercise intensity. (It's just like it sounds: you use body cues to perceive how you feel during an exercise.) Perceived exertion is a training intensity approach to HIIT training that I, and other certified exercise professionals around the world, have found to be a particularly safe and effective way for people of all fitness levels to enjoy HIIT. Also, every workout in this section can be adjusted from approximately 10 minutes to 20 minutes, as they are variable duration workouts. With these kinds of workouts, you adapt the length of your workout to your fitness level and/or daily fitness status. For instance, on some days you may want to train for 20 minutes, while on other days you may only have 10 minutes for your workout. For those of you who enjoy doing muscle strengthening exercises, in this section (in Chapter 21: The Future of HIIT Workouts—25 MORE Workouts!), I also introduce a very popular new training program called HIIT circuit training. These workouts combine the HIIT workouts with very popular muscular fitness circuit training for a fabulous total body workout you are sure to enjoy.

Finally, Section 4: 100 WINNING Ways to Cut Calories in Your Daily Life is my special gift to you. Here's why I call it a gift: in my numerous years of working with exercise devotees in the fitness world, one of the most common questions I get is, "what are ways I can cut calories in my daily life?" Many people don't want to jump into a new diet; they tried dieting and realized it just doesn't work for them. They are, however, still looking for ways to cut calories daily. Well, I've got the answer. I've gathered one hundred bona fide ways you can reduce calories on a daily basis. I am hoping you will find great enjoyment and personal satisfaction in seeing how daily smart tips to reduce calories will help you achieve and maintain weight management success. Are you ready to get started? Let's HIIT it!

Exercise, HIIT, and You

CHAPTER 1

Exercise: The Quality of Life Super Pill

WHEN I TRAVEL AROUND THE WORLD I AM OFTEN ASKED THE SAME SIMPLE QUESTION: WHY should I exercise? Let me explain it this way: Now more than ever, an abundance of evidence suggests that exercise is a super pill that is guaranteed to give its users a higher quality of life, needn't cost a penny, and doesn't come in a capsule. I will turn to my academic side to share with you the benefits of exercise, a topic I've written about extensively during my professional career.

Simply put, exercise and regular physical activity are considered a primary strategy for preventing, delaying, or combating numerous diseases. Interestingly, the importance of exercise for improving health was recognized by Hippocrates, the famous ancient Greek physician who wrote the following in the fifth century BC: "All parts of the body . . . if used in moderation and exercised in labors to which each is accustomed, become thereby healthy and well developed and age slowly; but if they are unused and left idle, they become liable to disease, defective in growth, and age quickly." This ancient wisdom was validated in 2012, when the journal *Comprehensive Physiology* published one of the most comprehensive scientific reviews on the benefits of exercise yet. This paper confirmed that regular physical activity and exercise are a primary prevention for thirty-five chronic diseases and health conditions. Some of the major health conditions that regular physical activity may combat include the following: coronary heart disease, type 2 diabetes (including prediabetes and gestational diabetes), obesity, metabolic syndrome (a group of risk factors including high blood pressure, high blood sugar, unhealthy high triglyceride levels, and abdominal fat), peripheral artery disease, hypertension, stroke, congestive heart failure, osteoporosis, osteoarthritis, bone fracture (and falls), rheumatoid arthritis, colon cancer, breast cancer, endometrial (uterus) cancer, accelerated aging, nonalcoholic fatty liver disease, constipation, gallbladder diseases, deep vein thrombosis, cognitive dysfunction, and depression. Yes, exercise can battle all of these diseases. In a 2016 article in the *British Journal of Sports Medicine*, the authors declare that exercise is just good medicine. I totally agree. And yet, despite these wondrous health benefits, most people do not exercise. As a result, American society continues to face major health challenges. Let me continue this story.

SITTING IS THE NEW SMOKING DISEASE

The 2012 *Comprehensive Physiology* article highlighted the fact that 95% of adults in the United States do not meet the minimum guideline for physical activity, which, as explained earlier, is 150 minutes of somewhat hard exercise throughout the week. Why is it such a struggle for the majority of Americans to attain 30 minutes of somewhat hard physical activity at least 5 days per week? Some scientists explain that there has been a steep decline in physical activity during the last several decades due to our reliance on technology, including automobiles, computers, televisions, smartphones, tablets, and energy-saving devices. Our new technologies have advanced travel, communication, education, research, business, and medicine, but have also contributed to a massive spike in physical inactivity (what we scientists refer to as "sedentary behavior"). People in developed societies throughout the world are spending greater amounts of time in activities that not only limit physical activity, but also require prolonged sitting. Schools, homes, worksites, and public spaces are built in ways to minimize human movement and promote sitting. When it comes to health, many wellness professionals now claim excessive sitting is akin to the smoking disease of yesteryear for its long-term health consequences.

Life is motion; we are a species designed to regularly move. Movement is vital for health and optimal aging. Accordingly, inspiring you to move more is a major goal of this book, and my START MOVING NOW! program, which is based on articles I've written, will help you combat sedentary behavior. My goal for most people I work with is to move more during their waking day. The benefits of this kind of lifestyle change are plain—and supported by research. In fact, a June 2016 article in the journal *Diabetes Care* showed that people who break up their waking days with movement are likely to reduce the risk of diabetes and cardiovascular complications. I encourage you to start moving more every day, and keep moving for the rest of your sure-to-be-vibrant life.

A NEW FITNESS TEAM IS FORMING

The medical community is now beginning to work closely with fitness professionals to help encourage people to get physically active. For its part, the American College of Sports Medicine has developed a new medical campaign promoting physical activity and exercise known as Exercise is Medicine (EIM). EIM is an international health initiative that encourages healthcare providers and primary care physicians to include physical activity when prescribing treatment plans for their patients. Many of these primary care physicians also refer their patients to credentialed exercise programs and certified exercise professionals. This collaboration between the medical community and fitness pros sends an invaluable message to everyone, regardless of their age: start moving, keep moving, and make exercise an essential part of your daily life. Remember, "Inch by inch, it's a cinch."

CHAPTER 2

What Is High-Intensity Interval Training (HIIT)?

I AM REGULARLY INVITED TO FITNESS CONFERENCES AROUND THE WORLD TO DISCUSS THE physiological merits of HIIT workouts and how to design HIIT programs. It is a big focus of my professional life, so I'd like to take this opportunity to explain it to you in more detail.

HIIT is a system of cardiovascular training that involves alternating between high- and light- intensity intervals of exercise of varying lengths of time. The high-intensity intervals (often referred to as work periods) may range from 5 seconds to 8 minutes long, and are performed at a self-regulated intensity ranging from comfortable-but-challenging to more challenging. The light-intensity intervals, called the recovery periods, are self-paced periods of exercise at a light-to-moderate intensity. When we speak of intensity, we are talking about the level of exercise exertion, or how hard you exercise. Each workout begins with a gradual warm-up that prepares the body for the following workout. This continues into the HIIT part of the workout, where alternating work and recovery intervals total a combined 10 to 20 minutes—or longer, if you are endurance-trained. Every HIIT workout concludes with a total body cooldown to return the body's heart rate, breathing rate, blood flow, and temperature back to a pre-exercise level.

In the book introduction I stated that true HIIT workouts are cardiovascular workouts. All of the wonderful health, disease prevention, and fat loss benefits are based on these types of workouts. Plus, all of the workouts in this book are adapted from actual studies that show these fabulous outcomes. Please note that the word "high-intensity" is a buzzword in the fitness industry for any workout that is very challenging. There are countless high-intensity workouts in the fitness industry (such as boot camp and body blast), however not all of them are actual HIIT programs.

WHY IS HIIT SO POPULAR?

Recently, interest in HIIT has grown enormously due to the widespread popularity of exercise programs, including P90X, Insanity, and CrossFit, all of which include aspects of HIIT. Millions of exercise buffs have found that alternating hard-intensity intervals of exercise with light-intensity intervals of recovery leads to enjoyable fitness gains in less time. In fact, in a 12-week 2017 study published in the *Journal of Diabetes Research*, it took obese sedentary women half the time to lose the same amount of body fat through HIIT training as it took them to lose it through traditional aerobic exercise. Another advantage of HIIT is the ease with which it can be modified for people of all fitness levels and health conditions. HIIT has generated a great deal of support with special populations, such as overweight individuals and those with clinical conditions like type 2 diabetes and cardiovascular disease. HIIT workouts can be performed with every kind of exercise modality, including cycling, walking, swimming, aqua training, elliptical striding, and in many group exercise classes. Also, HIIT workouts provide similar, and perhaps better, fitness benefits than continuous moderate-intensity aerobic workouts—what we call "steady-state workouts"—but in shorter periods of time.

Even more appealingly, HIIT workouts tend to burn more calories than traditional workouts, particularly after the workout; yes, that is correct—*after* the workout. Let me explain further. During the time period immediately following a workout, the body experiences an exercise "afterburn," or excess post-exercise oxygen consumption (EPOC) in exercise science terms. That's a mouthful, so let me put it in plain words. After every workout, your body's muscles and major systems, such as cardiovascular and respiratory, are still revved up. As a result, it takes energy to recover from exercise, and EPOC represents the energy expenditure you utilize to restore your body after your workout. So as you gradually slow down your muscles and return your body systems to pre-exercise levels, you continue to burn additional calories. This EPOC period tends to peak for about a 2-hour period after an exercise workout, though it may last up to 14 hours or longer. That means your metabolism is actually boosted for 2 or more hours after your workout.

Harder intensity workouts lead to longer EPOC periods. That's the impressive news about HIIT and EPOC, and why I wanted to highlight it here. Because of the dynamic nature of HIIT workouts, the EPOC periods tend to be longer than they are with traditional steady-state workouts. Therefore, HIIT workouts enable you to burn more calories. This additional calorie burn helps you achieve your weight management goals, which is another benefit of HIIT training highly praised by exercise aficionados.

Interestingly—and quite satisfyingly—during EPOC the body uses primarily fat to restore the body. So, a longer EPOC means the body is burning more fat after the workout, which is another plus from your HIIT workouts.

HOW ARE HIIT PROGRAMS DEVELOPED?

When you develop a HIIT program, you must consider the intensity (how hard you are exercising), the interval time ratio (length of work interval in relation to length of recovery interval), the workout duration (length of workout), and workout frequency (how many times a week). When it comes to deciding on an intensity, I recommend you use a rating system based on your perceived exertion during your workouts. Ratings of perceived exertion is a self-paced way for you to select the appropriate exercise intensity, and it's scientifically sound. For the work intervals, I encourage you to exercise at an intensity between comfortable-but-challenging and comfortable-but-more-challenging. These distinctions are entirely subjective; your senses will help you accurately and effectively gauge the intensity. You will use perceived exertion to self-monitor your workout intensity, and quite precisely. In fact, exercise enthusiasts, fitness professionals, and scientists have been using the perceived-exertion method to self-monitor exercise intensity for the last fifty years. For your recovery intervals, choose an exertion level that feels like a light-to-moderate intensity. (We'll discuss the details of the perceived exertion approach more thoroughly in Section 3, prior to starting the HIIT workouts.)

Another rather simple way to monitor your workout intensity is with the talk test. Using the talk test as your guide, a comfortable-but-challenging workout would be one where you are able to carry on a conversation, but have some difficulty speaking. I know it may seem a little bizarre, but there are studies that show the talk test is a very reliable measure of exercise intensity. Using the talk test as a guide, during the recovery intervals you should be able to carry on a conversation with mild to no difficulty.

When it comes to designing HIIT workouts, particularly those created by sports performance coaches, a major consideration is the time ratio between the work and recovery intervals. This time ratio describes the length of the work interval and the length of recovery interval. Essentially, this ratio can be deliberately designed to improve a specific sport performance variable. For instance, with track sprinters, coaches use short powerful work intervals to improve the speed and power of the athletes. Powerful bursts are followed by recovery intervals, which are often two to four times longer, to allow the athlete to fully recover. Many coaches use a specific time ratio of work intervals to recovery intervals to improve a specific energy system (such as the aerobic system) in their athletes. For example, a time ratio of 1 to 1, written 1:1, might be a 3-minute work (or high-intensity) interval followed by a 3-minute recovery (or light-intensity) interval. As you can see, 3 minutes of work and 3 minutes of recovery is a 1:1 ratio. Some of these 1:1 HIIT workouts often incorporate 3-, 4-, or 5-minute work intervals alternately, followed by of recovery intervals of an equal length of time.

These 1:1 time ratio workouts seem to be very good for endurance athletes and help them perform better in their endurance competitions. Here's another example that illustrates the use of strategically designed intervals. There's a popular HIIT training protocol called the "sprint interval training method." With this type of program, the person exercising does up to 30 seconds of sprinting effort for the work intervals, followed by recovery intervals ranging from 30 seconds up to 4.5 minutes. I include several sprint interval workouts in this book.

In regard to workout duration, HIIT workouts may last from 5 minutes to approximately 60 minutes. For those of you using this book, I have designed the HIIT workouts to be from 10–20 minutes as this has been shown to be highly effective and time efficient. The duration of the workout is influenced by a person's fitness level and goals. When looking at the duration of a HIIT workout, we do not traditionally count the warm-up or cooldown minutes to determine the length of the HIIT workout. So, if you did ten 30-second work intervals alternating with ten recovery intervals, each 30 seconds long, we would just say the entire HIIT workout is 10 minutes.

Frequency of HIIT workouts is our last consideration in designing HIIT workouts. HIIT workouts may be more exhausting than steady-state workouts (which are usually completed at a continuous low-to-moderate intensity during the entire workout), and therefore, a longer period of rest is often needed between them. Perhaps start with two HIIT training workouts a week, with any other aerobic workouts being steady-state workouts, such as brisk walking, cycling, swimming. When you feel ready for a greater challenge, increase your workout frequency by adding a third HIIT workout a week. It is best not to do HIIT workouts on back-to-back days, though. Try to spread your HIIT workouts throughout the week.

MAXIMIZE YOUR RESULTS AND MINIMIZE THE RISKS WITH HIIT

Most importantly, regardless of your age, gender, and fitness level, safe participation and enjoyment of HIIT workouts (and all exercise programs for that matter) requires that you adjust the intensity of the workout to your preferred challenge level. When it comes to exercise, safety should always be your number one priority. Focus first on finding your own optimal training intensity, not just keeping up with other people. Some fitness leaders promote the idea that you have to exercise at an all-out intensity level for the HIIT workout to be beneficial—this is not correct. In fact, I suggest you avoid exercising at an all-out intensity during your workouts. Pushing yourself to this level may potentially cause bodily harm. In *HIIT Your Limit!*, the recurring message is that you should exercise at a comfortable-but-challenging to more challenging intensity during your HIIT work intervals. There is a big difference between a healthy challenge workout and one that is too difficult. So, comfortable-but-challenging is your goal when doing the harder (work) intervals in your HIIT workouts. You can do it!

CHAPTER 3

What Are the Health Benefits of HIIT?

HIIT IS AN APPROACH TO EXERCISE TRAINING THAT PROVIDES MANY HEALTH AND FITNESS benefits in a notably time-efficient manner. Numerous studies have been conducted and published about the effects of this unique form of training on different populations, such as athletes, healthy men and women enthusiasts, obese people, and individuals with disease. In this section I am going to highlight HIIT research as it relates to cardiorespiratory fitness, cholesterol levels, blood pressure, and weight management. Things get a bit technical in this part of this book, but bear with me. I really want you to realize how healthy this exercise program may be for you!

HOW MUCH CAN HIIT IMPROVE CARDIORESPIRATORY FITNESS?

Cardiorespiratory fitness, also called aerobic fitness, refers to the ability of the heart, blood vessels, and lungs to supply oxygen-rich blood to exercising muscle tissues and the ability of the muscles to use the supplied oxygen to produce energy for a workout. That's a lot to absorb in one sentence, so let's break it down: cardiorespiratory fitness is a measure of your ability to consume oxygen, deliver it to your exercising muscles, and take and use the oxygen for energy production. Hopefully this makes better sense.

When it comes to improving cardiorespiratory fitness, HIIT is a marvel. In a comprehensive 2011 review in the *Journal of Obesity*, it was reported that healthy young and older adult men and women can improve their cardiorespiratory fitness up to 46% after 8 to 15 weeks of HIIT training. For the record, that is a staggering improvement in a relatively short period of time. Of course, the degree of improvement a person will actually achieve is directly related to her/his fitness level. For instance, the lower a person's baseline fitness level, the greater the gains she/he will potentially make in cardiorespiratory fitness. Thus, individuals who lead sedentary lifestyles and then begin an exercise program will likely see the largest gains in cardiorespiratory fitness with a progressive and consistent training program. Conversely, people who have been regularly training for years will have smaller, incremental gains that are clearly not as large as those made by their sedentary counterparts.

According to current scientific research, this impressively swift increase in cardiorespiratory fitness is due to a major improvement in the heart's blood pumping capacity, referred to as "stroke volume." Stroke volume is the amount of blood pumped by the heart each heartbeat. Your heart, which is the size of your fist, pumps blood through its heart chambers in a way similar to how you quickly clench and open your fist. And, as the heart gets stronger, it pumps stronger, ejecting more blood (i.e., stroke volume) with each heartbeat.

Your ability to sustain aerobic exercise depends on your heart's ability to continually pump oxygen-rich blood to the working muscles. The oxygen is needed to harvest the energy compound that powers movement, ATP. In fact, the presence of oxygen in the body's cells actually boosts all of the major cell reactions that lead to the formation of ATP. So, the more oxygen present at the exercising muscle, the longer your muscles can last during the workout. Simply put, a stronger heart pumps more blood carrying oxygen to the working muscles.

Another fascinating cardiorespiratory adaptation of the body—one well observed during HIIT workouts—can be seen in your muscles. Your muscles move your body and are fueled by incredible bean-shaped, energy-producing organelles known as "mitochondria." Mitochondria are often referred to as the energy factories of your cells. Depending on a person's training and genetics, each individual muscle cell may have four hundred to two thousand of these powerhouse mitochondria. With regular HIIT workouts, mitochondria get bigger and the body makes more of them in the muscle cells. Isn't that amazing? This occurrence is seen in women and men of all ages, fitness levels, and ethnic backgrounds. Therefore, the size and number of mitochondria directly translates into enhanced cardiorespiratory fitness at any level of exercise intensity.

From a health perspective, this cardiorespiratory improvement is invaluable, because low aerobic fitness is directly linked to heart attack and other health-related causes of mortality. In a large, 1996 pioneering study at the famous Cooper Institute in Dallas, Texas, researchers studied the medical exams and cardiorespiratory tests of 25,341 men and 7,080 women. The results of this landmark study indicated that adults who are moderately or highly fit had enhanced cardioprotection. "Cardioprotection" is a relatively new term in science. It means those women and men who were fitter had better defenses against heart disease and heart attacks, compared to women and men who were less fit. This finding was found to be true regardless of whether the individuals were smokers or nonsmokers, had normal or elevated cholesterol levels, or were obese or had average body weights. Another prominent study, this one published in the *American Journal of Cardiology* in 2006, concurs with the results of the Cooper Institute investigation. In this study, the researchers found that vigorous exercise intensity was more beneficial (i.e., more cardioprotective) in positively altering one or more risk factors to heart disease.

What do these results tell us? They remind us that regular HIIT workouts should be considered to be among the most effective ways of counteracting the effects of heart disease, the number one cause of death throughout the world. Here's your take-home message: Keep striving to incrementally improve your cardiorespiratory fitness. The fitter your heart and lungs, the healthier and better equipped you are to fight off disease. As the old saying goes, keep moving briskly for enhanced cardioprotection!

WHAT IS THE EFFECT OF HIIT ON INSULIN SENSITIVITY?

The term "insulin sensitivity" refers to the ability of the muscles to successfully utilize glucose for fuel. Insulin works very much like a key in a doorknob: it helps to unlock transporter proteins that bring glucose into the muscles for fuel. So, having high insulin sensitivity is very healthy, because it means insulin is working effectively to help bring glucose into the muscles. Several research teams have investigated the effect of HIIT on improving insulin sensitivity. Taken together, the results indicate that HIIT can increase insulin sensitivity by 23% to 58%. That is quite impressive! This great news means that HIIT training increases the ability of your body to take up glucose into the muscle cells to use for energy. This helps to prevent high blood glucose levels, a precursor to type 2 diabetes. Studies show this increase in insulin sensitivity begins around week two of your training and progressively improves over the next 16 weeks of your HIIT workouts. Your body rapidly adapts to your new exercise program by more effectively taking up glucose from the blood.

The reason for this improvement in insulin sensitivity from HIIT training is well understood. Scientists have discovered that exercising your muscles actually activates the body's glucose transporter proteins, called "GLUT4 proteins." Your HIIT workouts prompt these proteins to take glucose into the muscles for fuel.

You may be asking: why is this important? Here's why. Under normal conditions, your muscles use insulin to activate the GLUT4 proteins to take glucose into the muscles (as explained). However, for people with insulin resistance, also called low insulin sensitivity, and type 2 diabetes, insulin is not able to effectively stimulate these GLUT4 proteins. What does this mean in real-world terms? It tells us that HIIT workouts are an excellent line of defense toward the prevention and/or management of type 2 diabetes, one of the fastest growing diseases throughout the world.

WHAT IS THE EFFECT OF HIIT ON CHOLESTEROL LEVELS?

Cholesterol is a waxy, fat-like substance that's found in all cells of the body. One of its most important functions is to aid in the production of hormones, and it also plays a chief role in constructing our cell membranes. It's transported in the blood by special protein packages called "lipoproteins." The two most important lipoproteins to know about are low-density lipoproteins (LDL) and high-density lipoproteins (HDL). LDL cholesterol is often called the "lousy" cholesterol because an excess of LDL in the blood builds up on the artery walls, creating the plaque that leads to heart disease. On the flip side, HDL cholesterol is frequently called good or healthy cholesterol because it's responsible for removing and transporting cholesterol from the artery walls to the liver, where it is disposed of by the body. Having an elevated level of HDL is believed to be favorably associated with preventing heart disease, that is, having enhanced cardioprotection.

In 2012, an article in the journal *Sports Medicine* reviewed fourteen studies that examined the effect of HIIT workouts on cholesterol levels. The researchers found that HIIT has been shown to elevate your body's "good" (HDL) cholesterol in as little as 8 weeks of training. This is excellent news, considering that HDL cholesterol helps clear out the dangerous plaque that accumulates on the inside of arteries and blood vessels. Increased levels of HDL cholesterol mean your blood has more plaque-devouring scavengers to help get rid of risky plaque build-up. In addition, the scientists who conducted the study believe that HIIT workouts, in combination with a decrease in body fat (or body weight), lower the "lousy" (LDL) cholesterol and other circulating blood fats in your blood. To summarize, there is solid evidence that HIIT workouts are a direct line of defense in combatting heart disease.

WHAT IS THE EFFECT OF HIIT ON BLOOD PRESSURE?

Additionally, the same 2012 article in *Sports Medicine* concluded people with elevated blood pressure (who were not on any hypertension medicine) positively and appreciably lowered their blood pressure after at least 12 weeks of HIIT training. The research shows that progressive and consistent HIIT workouts may lower systolic and diastolic blood pressure by about 2% to 8%—no small deal. As you may know, systolic blood pressure measures the pressure on your heart when it is ejecting blood and diastolic blood pressure measures it when your heart is refilling with blood. Left untreated for years, elevated blood pressure increases your risk of heart attack and heart failure. Over time, the strain on the heart caused by high blood pressure weakens your heart muscle, causing it to lose pumping strength, and the higher blood pressure damages the inner linings of arteries. It literally scrapes away on the crucial linings of arteries, causing the arteries to lose their elasticity. You want your arteries to be flexible and able to stretch; if they are not able to, your blood circulation will be impeded. HIIT workouts help to counteract high blood pressure and keep your arteries flexible.

HOW DOES HIIT IMPACT FAT LOSS AND WEIGHT MANAGEMENT?

There are many ways in which HIIT workouts help reduce body fat and promote healthy weight management goals. In the previously referenced 2011 research review published in the *Journal of Obesity*, it was found that HIIT workouts cause a striking surge in epinephrine and norepinephrine, also known as adrenaline and noradrenaline, respectively. Adrenaline and noradrenaline are your fight-or-flight hormones. These hormones are also known to ignite the breakdown or burning of fat by your exercising muscles. In addition, the surge of fight-or-flight hormones stimulates fat cells to release some of the body's stored fat, which then becomes fuel for exercise. A 2017 study in the *Journal of Diabetes Research* also found that HIIT workouts have the potential to help reduce your abdominal fat stores, a process that has positive health implications. Fat around the middle of the body is highly associated with the development of heart disease and type 2 diabetes, so gradually depleting this abdominal fat is an important step in reducing a major health risk. Plus, reducing abdominal fat is one of the most common goals for people trying to improve their health and fitness.

I am often asked, and you are probably wondering, how long does it take for your body to start improving its fat burning capabilities from HIIT workouts? In a 2007 study published in the *Journal of Applied Physiology*, researchers determined that moderately active women in the study significantly improved their muscles' fat burning capacity in as little as seven HIIT training sessions spread out over 2 weeks. This is a remarkable finding, and one definitely worth repeating for emphasis: *it took subjects only 2 weeks and seven HIIT workouts to significantly improve their fat-burning capability*. This is compelling evidence that HIIT training helps the body rapidly improve its fat-burning capacity. Combined with a sound weight management plan, HIIT training can be the key to optimal weight loss. (A comprehensive, state-of-the art weight management plan is provided in the second section of the book.)

SUMMARY OF THE MAJOR HEALTH BENEFITS OF HIIT

Without a doubt, improvement in cardiorespiratory fitness is one of the most life-changing benefits of HIIT workouts. This improvement is directly related to enhanced cardioprotection from heart disease and a number of other health enhancements, such as improving insulin sensitivity. HIIT workouts stimulate GLUT4 proteins, helping the body better utilize blood sugar and keep it from rising, which in turn helps prevent type 2 diabetes (or, helps diabetics better manage it). Also, HIIT's effect on fat loss and fat utilization are particularly encouraging, as is the impact of HIIT on reducing systolic and diastolic blood pressure (when elevated) and improving HDL cholesterol. The evidence is in, and it shows that HIIT is a health-packed winner workout for all. Let's keep moving, people!

CHAPTER 4

How Does Your Body Power Your HIIT Workouts?

AS YOU LAUNCH FORWARD INTO THE MANY HIIT WORKOUTS IN THIS BOOK, I REALLY WANT you to understand how your body remarkably responds and adapts to these workouts. Even though I am an exercise physiologist, I am still totally amazed by the human body, particularly during exercise. As a result, I wish to share with you a glimpse of my world, my fellow HIIT enthusiasts (or soon-to-be enthusiasts!)—the world that studies what happens to the body when you exercise. In this short chapter, I hope you become just as enthralled with your body's proficiency as I am.

INTRODUCING ATP, THE FUEL FOR LIFE AND EXERCISE

To power your exercise and daily life activities, your body relies for energy on a chemical compound called "adenosine triphosphate," or just ATP (discussed briefly in the previous chapter). ATP is produced when your body's cells disassemble carbohydrates and fats from the foods you eat. To disassemble *fat*, our body must use quite a bit of oxygen, which is where we get the name "aerobic energy system." In contrast, your cells can disassemble carbohydrates with or without oxygen present. When the cells do this without oxygen, we call it the "anaerobic energy system."

Students always ask me, what about the proteins? Don't proteins provide a lot of energy for exercise? Actually, proteins are used only sparingly for fuel during exercise. Here's why: the proteins you eat are digested and broken down into specific amino acids. Most of these amino acids are used to make new proteins, which build and repair muscles, tissues, skin, and bones; other amino acids help make hormones and messenger chemicals for the body. What amino acids don't do, however, is power a workout.

The deep involvement of the body's two energy systems, aerobic and anaerobic, is part of what makes HIIT workouts so unique. Let's journey a little deeper into these systems.

THE AEROBIC ENERGY SYSTEM: THE LONG-TERM ENERGY SOURCE

The aerobic energy system is the chief energy production system of the body, and the most efficient one. The term aerobic literally means "with oxygen." As the name implies, this energy system cannot work unless there is sufficient oxygen available in the muscles during exercise. It takes about 5 minutes to fully turn on the pathways for the aerobic energy system to provide enough ATP for the workout. In other words, your aerobic system needs a brief start-up period before it provides enough ATP for your muscles to complete a sustained HIIT workout.

Your aerobic energy system capacity is primarily dependent on your training status. Perhaps this is best illustrated during the Olympics, when we see world champion athletes accomplishing magnificent endurance feats at the world's most competitive level. This is a spot-on example of the colossal potential of the human body to adapt to high-quality training. I tell my students that your aerobic energy system is analogous to a large double-decker bus with a hefty gas tank. Modern buses can travel at relatively moderate speeds for great lengths of time. Similarly, via the aerobic energy system, we can tap into our carbohydrate and fat reserves for fuel, and with the help of oxygen your body can exercise for long periods at light, moderate, or hard intensities. During prolonged workouts such as cycling, cross-country skiing, and distance running, your muscles are dependent on the aerobic energy system's ability to continuously produce ATP. In my exercise science classes we call the aerobic energy system "mitochondrial respiration."

Let's break down the term, mitochondrial respiration. First, as you may recall from your earlier reading in the book, mitochondria are small, bean-shaped organelles in your cells. They are the energy factories that completely disassemble fats and carbohydrates, and with the help of oxygen, produce the ATP needed for sustained aerobic exercise (and life). The term "respiration" refers simply to the use of oxygen in the aerobic energy system.

My students often ask me why our bodies don't exclusively use fats for fuel in mitochondrial respiration. They pose their question like this: we store so much more fat than carbohydrates, so why don't we use 100% fat for fuel for exercise? Here's my answer: during exercise, our need for ATP is massive; we need it to keep us moving. And, as discussed above, the source of ATP is fats and carbohydrates. Our cells break down fats for fuel much more slowly than they break down carbohydrates, so, as our need for energy increases during high-intensity workouts such as HIIT, our muscle cells call on carbohydrates to come to the rescue. We are always burning fats during exercise, but as our intensity increases we use quite a bit of carbohydrates too, because they can produce ATP quite fast. The great news is, the more regularly you do HIIT workouts, the faster your body learns how to burn fat to make ATP. So, one of the greatest benefits of regular aerobic exercise is that it trains your muscles to become very efficient fat-burning engines.

THE ANAEROBIC ENERGY SYSTEM: THE SOURCE OF RAPID ENERGY

Anaerobic literally means "without oxygen." The anaerobic energy system is activated during activities requiring quick bursts of energy, such as lifting weights, running short races, jumping, and throwing. The anaerobic energy system will also be called on to help the aerobic system during the work intervals in your HIIT workouts. Essentially, you are going to power your challenging HIIT work intervals with your aerobic *and* anaerobic energy systems working as a team. Together they will give you the ATP fuel you need to exercise.

THE MUSCLES ARE THE ENGINES THAT DO THE WORK

Finally, we'll complete the story of how the body powers your HIIT workouts with an overview of muscles. Muscles are of great interest to exercise enthusiasts and scientists (and beachgoers, too). Your muscles attach to the skeleton and contract continuously during exercise. Muscles are powered by ATP, which comes from the aerobic and anaerobic energy systems. Your bones provide the structure for the muscles to do their work, enabling your body to move. Think of muscles as the engines driving your body's movements and the skeleton as a complex arrangement of levers, fulcrums, and force arms that carry out the movements. As you continue to challenge the muscles of your body, they rapidly learn and adapt to work harder and function better. Regularly doing HIIT workouts is going to lead to a healthier, stronger you. Let's keep going!

CHAPTER 5

Ten Steps to Succeed in an Exercise Program

ONE OF THE BIGGEST CHALLENGES WITH ANY EXERCISE PROGRAM IS STICKING TO IT. Movement is natural, but exercise is a unique behavior that we all have to learn. As you start exercising, don't let early awkwardness or uneven skill development get you down—it happens to everyone. In fact, you will be amazed by how fast you learn and adapt to exercise effectively and capably. To help you become a steadfast exercise enthusiast, I devised the following ten steps on how to succeed in an exercise program. They are drawn from the scientific literature and my many years in the fitness industry.

1. **SET GOALS BEFORE YOU BEGIN.** Having short-term and long-term goals makes a big difference. For fitness goal setting, think of your short-term goals as daily, weekly, or even monthly targets, and consider your long-term goals as semiannual and/or annual ones. Do you remember the philosophical approach I follow when working with fitness, health, and weight management enthusiasts (the philosophy I presented in the book's introduction)? Yes, it's the phrase, "Inch by inch, it's a cinch." To apply this approach to yourself, break up your goals into manageable stages. Also, as you progress in your exercise program, feel free to revisit and modify your goals at any time. You are ready. To help you stay on track, I invite you to write out a personal fitness contract for yourself that answers these goal-oriented questions:

a) What is one overall (and major) long-term goal of your exercise program you'd like to achieve in the next 6 months? Would you like to lose some weight? If yes, how much weight per month for the next 6 months?

b) What are some short-term goals you'd like to attain on a daily and weekly basis? Think this through and then answer these questions: Do you want to be active each week? If so, how many days per week would you like to do some physical activity? How many minutes per day would you like to exercise? Do you want to join a fitness facility or sign up for an exercise class? If so, when do you want this to begin? Do you want to eat more of a heart-healthy diet? Go ahead, write down all of these short-term goals.

After you've done this, evaluate your goals and determine the best way to manage and organize your plan of action. Sometimes it helps to schedule a meeting with a certified fitness professional to discuss your goals. If this is not an option, you may wish to choose a close friend who you feel will help you achieve success. Ask this person to read your goals and provide sincere, constructive, nonjudgmental feedback. Finally, both of you should sign your personal contract when it is complete. It helps when you commit yourself to your goals and have the other person sign, too, because this shows you are accountable to this person.

2. **REWARD YOURSELF AS YOU ATTAIN SOME OF YOUR GOALS.** Keep track of your progress. As you achieve some of the goals you have written out in your fitness contract, reward yourself with a thoughtful gift, such as a book, new outfit, movie, new app, show, or—better yet—some new exercise gear.

3. **REGULARLY SELF-EVALUATE HOW YOUR EXERCISE PROGRAM (AND LIFESTYLE) IS PROGRESSING.** To evaluate your progress, I suggest you write (or type) out a health, fitness, and lifestyle evaluation list that includes things you are doing right (such as not smoking, eating well, and not abusing substances) and things you need to improve (such as not consistently exercising, neglecting to deal with stress, and sleeping inconsistently). Next, self-assess ways you can shift more entries to the "right" side. For instance, learning

some yoga breathing techniques may help you manage your stress and improve your sleep patterns. Self-evaluation is a great way to consistently self-improve.

4. **FIND A WORKOUT PARTNER.** Research on sticking to an exercise program indicates we are more likely to adhere to daily exercise routines when we exercise with another person or persons. It's best to partner with someone whose fitness level and goals are similar to yours (but if that's not possible, any partner who gives you support for your exercise program is still better than no partner). Discuss what exercise activities or fitness classes you both enjoy, and commit to participating in them as workout partners.

5. **SCHEDULE YOUR WORKOUTS ON YOUR DAILY AND MONTHLY CALENDAR.** With your workout partner, schedule your exercise sessions 3 to 5 days per week. Treat your workout time like a special meeting that can't be cancelled (except for emergencies), because doing so will help ensure you don't just blow it off for other obligations and tasks. I am frequently asked if it is better to exercise in the early morning, mid-morning, afternoon, or evening. My reply is always the same: select a time of day that has the best chance of helping you succeed. And if you discover the time you've chosen doesn't seem to work, feel empowered to try another time. Let's face it: you, like most people, are juggling multiple work-related and family-related activities daily. Once you determine a time or times that are best for your workouts, be selfish about preserving that time for your workouts. Dedicate this time block to yourself.

6. **GET IN TUNE WITH YOUR BODY BY "BODY CHECKING."** Body checking is a technique I have used with my students for many years, and something you can do readily. Let me explain how it works. Always assess how your body reacts during your workout and recovers after your workout. If something feels too hard, immediately slow down or lighten the intensity. If it feels too easy, go ahead and challenge yourself a little more. If you are unusually tired after your workouts, you are most likely doing too much, or your diet is insufficient to fuel your workouts. Body checking is a way of listening to your bodily signals during and after exercise and then responding to them. I call it "body checking" because your body is incredibly intelligent, and during exercise it is sending you hundreds of signals. Listen to these

messages and respond appropriately! If you are just starting a new exercise program, such as your HIIT workouts, it is always best to progress gradually. Over the years I've always told students and clients I've trained that the first several workouts should feel too easy. Let your body adjust to the workouts and build strength and stamina. Most fitness injuries come from people doing too much, too soon, too fast, and too hard; don't get trapped in this downward spiral, as it may lead to your early "retirement" from exercise. Learning body checking shows a real dedication to respecting your exercising body.

7. **WEAR COMFORTABLE CLOTHING AND PROPER SHOES.** Your exercise clothing should permit you to move freely and allow your body to cool itself. Be aware that some exercise clothing fabrics have chemicals that may not be safe during exercise. Avoid exercise gear with acrylic, rayon, acetate, and stain-resistant chemicals (such as those treated with per-fluorinated chemicals). Some of the more exercise friendly fabrics include bamboo pulp, cotton, cotton blends, nylon, polyester, and spandex. Proper attire is important for exercise enjoyment and success. (In Chapter 16 we'll discuss workout gear and shoes further.)

8. **PLAN TO EXERCISE AT LEAST 1 TO 2 HOURS AFTER A MEAL.** By waiting to work out after eating a meal, you will prevent stomach cramping and pain. Eating too close to exercise may also make you too tired; you don't want your digestive system competing with your muscles for energy. Prior to a workout, always choose foods that your body finds easy to digest.

9. **BE READY FOR SOME EXERCISE SPEED BUMPS.** Yes, we all have speed bumps when it comes to exercise—even people who have been training for years. Most of these come in the form of a missed workout or a lapsed goal. First and foremost, don't get angry with yourself if you miss a workout or backslide on one of your goals. In fact, the first step is to forgive yourself for the lapse. Next, try to focus on what caused the lapse and how you may better deal with it in the future. For instance, if you start missing your workouts, perhaps you are scheduling them at the wrong time. Or, if you are too tired to exercise, it may be that you need to have a light snack a couple hours before your workout. Speed bumps are challenging, but *they won't* undo all the progress you've made. Take a moment, reflect, and focus on the best way(s) for getting back on track.

10. **CONSIDER USING A FITNESS TRACKER.** Our world is flourishing with fitness trackers, mobile apps, and other wearable devices that calculate our daily movements and exercise. Some of the newer fitness products are quite accurate in measuring calories, steps, heart rate, and other physiological data. These fitness trackers really do inspire people to move more. In 2007, a comprehensive study published in the *Journal of the American Medical Association* involved reviewing twenty-six previous studies in which participants used pedometers to increase their physical activity, and it found that the average increase in physical activity among participants was 2,491 steps per day, a 26.9% increase. Don't, however, expect trackers to help you automatically lose weight. Weight management, which I have dedicated the second section of this book to, requires learning new strategies to modify behaviors. Fitness trackers do not prompt you to change a behavior; they just track your activity, inspiring you to be more active. So consider trying a few of them out and seeing how they work for you. Most important is to stay positive and believe in yourself. You are in control.

Do It Right: Avoid These Exercise Mistakes

I WANT YOU TO REALLY ENJOY YOUR WORKOUTS. IF YOU DON'T, THERE'S A CHANCE YOU may make a mistake. To help you identify exercise mistakes and avoid them in the future, I'd like to provide some preventative guidance. Following it will help ensure that you don't harm yourself through your exercise program. Here are the seven most common exercise mistakes I have observed from my many years of exercise training and teaching.

1. **OVERTRAINING: IN THEIR PASSION TO ACHIEVE THEIR FITNESS GOALS, SOME PEOPLE TRY TOO HARD.** Enthusiasm is a wonderful thing, but taxing your body too much will not get you any closer to your goals. Possible signs of overtraining include injury, weight loss, mental dullness, disturbed digestion, loss of appetite, early exhaustion during a workout, fatigue during the day, and elevated heart rate (usually five to ten beats faster) upon awakening in the morning. If you experience any of these signs of overtraining, you may need to ease the intensity of your workouts and the duration of your total exercise time. Also, I realize that in order to achieve your desired health and weight management goals you may decide to limit your caloric intake while embarking on your HIIT training program. If so, make sure you maintain a healthy balance of carbohydrates, fats, and proteins in your three daily primary meals (and snacks).

2. **POOR EXERCISE TECHNIQUE.** Good technique in exercise means a person is doing an exercise that maximizes correct movement, and also minimizes the chances of injury. With good exercise movement technique, the body works together as a unit, rather than as a stockpile of parts.

   Poor technique is most likely to occur during the latter stages of a workout, when fatigue is starting to set in. This may put excessive pressure on your joints or muscles, thereby contributing to an injury. A good example of this is tennis elbow, which is often caused by having poor backhand technique. Another example is misusing a treadmill: holding onto the safety bars while running can negatively affect your posture and lead to knee, hip, shoulder, and back discomfort. When I teach someone a movement, I always encourage them to focus on its correct execution. The benefits of this attentive focus will carry over to your daily activities, such as lifting groceries, climbing stairs, rising from a chair, or running to catch a train or bus. So make a point to always emphasize quality in your workout movements and watch your daily activities improve too.

3. **IMPROPER EQUIPMENT.** The exercise clothes you wear, the shoes on your feet, the surface you are training on, and the equipment you are using can all improve or impair your performance. For those of you exercising at home, make sure you have plenty of space and ventilation for your exercise equipment and for you. Also, be aware of any safety concerns with the equipment you are using. For instance, treadmills are often identified as potentially dangerous pieces of fitness equipment. While the treadmill is in operation, its belt is constantly moving, and quite quickly. A fall can lead to abrasions, broken bones or sprained joints. That said, one of the leading contributors to treadmill injuries is simply inattention, so if you say focused you will minimize any risk of injury. The treadmill is not the place to check your phone, text, or conduct any activity other than walking or running.

4. **INSUFFICIENT WARM-UP: TOO OFTEN, THE MAIN WORKOUT IS STARTED WITHOUT PROPER WARM-UP OR AFTER A QUICK, INSUFFICIENT WARM-UP.** An appropriate warm-up progressively prepares your muscles, nerves, heart, and lungs for the challenging workout to follow. It also activates your mobility, coordination, and balance, getting you ready for the

dynamic movements in the workout. Note that the most effective warm-ups are tailored to the specific movements you will be doing during your main workout, since this prepares the muscles that will be used. So, if you will be biking during your HIIT workout, the best warm-up will be a bike warm-up. If you are rowing during your HIIT workout, then go ahead and row for your warm-up. Most warm-ups should start at a relatively light intensity and progress for 5 to 7 minutes.

5. **EXERCISES THAT ARE TOO BOUNCY AND FAST.** Movements that are too fast and bouncy stimulate opposing muscle groups to contract and hinder each movement. You want some of your movements to be dynamic, particularly during HIIT workouts—but not to the point where you are stressing your joints. I tell clients that movement speeds regularly vary in exercise. That is normal. However, focus more on moving with a controlled effort than the speed of your movement. That's the key!

6. **INADEQUATE COOLDOWN.** After your HIIT workout, it's time to do your cooldown. The cooldown is a progressive slowing of your exercise movements, and it helps to gradually lower your heart rate, breathing rate, and blood pressure toward pre-exercise levels. A successful cooldown helps to avoid fainting or dizziness, which can happen when blood remains in the large muscles of the legs. You want to keep the major muscles working slowly during the cooldown. The cooldown promotes blood flow back to the heart, where it is sent to the lungs to be loaded with fresh oxygen, and then sent to all of your body's major organs. At the end of your HIIT workouts perform a 3–5 minute cooldown, such as easy walking at a light intensity.

6. **REPEATING THE SAME EXACT WORKOUT.** Many people find a workout they enjoy and just keep doing it. However, in order to improve your health and fitness level, you need to continually challenge your body by doing a different workout, changing the intensity of your workout, or changing some components of your workouts. One of the problems with doing the same exact workout all the time is that your body adapts so readily it expends fewer and fewer calories to complete the workout; in science we say this increases your metabolic efficiency. But worry not—there are plenty of HIIT workouts in this book. I encourage you to enjoy them all!

7. **EXERCISING WHEN YOU ARE ILL.** Oftentimes, people who are serious about training may attempt to "exercise through" an illness (like a cold or flu), only to prolong their symptoms or cause a recurrence. This may further delay your return to exercising at an optimum level. It's always best to check in with your health practitioner to discuss and resolve any health issues you might have.

Time for Your Heart Health Pre-Check

I'D LIKE TO INTRODUCE YOU TO THE HEART HEALTH PRE-CHECK. THIS IS A SPECIAL HEALTH assessment to determine your risk for cardiovascular disease (CVD), the leading cause of death for women and men throughout the United States and the world. To assess your own CVD risk, I encourage you—again!—to contact your health practitioner, always a good idea before embarking on any program of strenuous exercise. Your practitioner will be able to give you the information you need to complete your heart health pre-check. But first, let's explore a little more about cardiovascular disease.

Cardiovascular disease is a term that encompasses diseases of the heart and blood vessels, coronary artery disease, heart attack, and stroke. A 2017 report by the American Heart Association found that CVD accounted for 801,000 deaths in the United States in the previous year. That means one in every three deaths in the US is due to CVD—a sobering statistic. As a result, identifying risk factors for CVD is vital to avoiding heart problems. A risk factor is anything that makes someone susceptible to a condition or illness; thus, a *positive* CVD risk factor is something that promotes CVD. A *negative* CVD risk factor is something that negates a positive CVD risk factor. (Contrary to what its name implies, a negative risk factor offers a health *advantage*.) This will be easier to understand as we go over the risk factors below.

Below is your heart health pre-check of positive CVD risk factors. Go over this with your health practitioner to better determine if you have any of these risk factors.

1. **FAMILY HISTORY OF HEART ATTACK.** This would be a heart attack or sudden death before fifty-five years of age in your father (or male first-degree relative, which means your parents, offspring, or siblings) or before sixty-five years of age in your mother (or female first-degree relative).

2. **CIGARETTE SMOKING.** Are you a current smoker or did you just quit within the last 6 months? If yes, this is a positive risk factor.

3. **HIGH BLOOD PRESSURE.** Is your systolic blood pressure ≥130 mmHg and/or is your diastolic blood pressure ≥80 mmHg? And if so, has this been confirmed on two separate occasions? Or, are you taking an antihypertensive medication? Answering yes to either of these questions means you are at risk.

4. **ABNORMAL CHOLESTEROL LEVELS.** Is your total cholesterol >200 mg/dL? Is your high-density (good) cholesterol <40 mg/dL? Are you on a lipid-lowering medication? Is your low-density (bad) cholesterol >130 mg/dL? If you can answer yes to at least one of these questions, you have this positive risk factor.

5. **PREDIABETES.** Is your fasting blood glucose ≥100 mg/dL and ≤125 mg/dL, and has this been confirmed on at least two separate occasions? If yes, this would be a positive risk factor.

6. **OBESITY.** Is your body mass index (BMI) ≥30 kg/m², or waist girth ≥40 inches for men and ≥35 inches for women? Answering yes to any of these means you are at risk.

7. **SEDENTARY LIFESTYLE.** Have you been participating in at least 30 minutes of moderate-intensity (somewhat hard) physical activity at least 3 days a week for the last 3 months? If not, this would be a positive risk factor.

8. **AGE.** Men, if you are forty-five years or older, this is a positive risk factor. Ladies, if you are fifty-five years or older, this is a positive risk factor.

There is only one negative risk factor, which means it negates a positive risk factor: elevated high-density lipoprotein cholesterol (HDL-C). Is your high-density lipoprotein cholesterol (HDL-C) >60 mg/dL? Since this is the good cholesterol, we would like for this value to be above 60 mg/dL. Having high HDL-C indicates this "scavenger" is cleaning up the plaque on your arteries, which is a great health benefit in the prevention of CVD.

Before we move on, let's quickly discuss how to interpret these CVD risk factors. For example, if a person is sedentary but has no other positive risk factors, we would say she/he has one positive risk factor. If this person also has an HDL-C of 65mg/dL (which is >60mg/dL) this person also has one negative risk factor. Therefore, in this example, the HDL-C negates the sedentary behavior risk. Having HDL-C >60 mg/dL will negate any *one* of the positive risk factors—but not all of them. Your goal is to have as few of the positive risk factors as possible.

You will not necessarily develop CVD if you have a positive risk factor. Nevertheless, the more positive risk factors you have, the greater the likelihood that you will get CVD at some point in your life. I highly encourage you to adopt a heart-healthy lifestyle in an effort to lower your CVD risk. Here are the key elements of a heart-healthy lifestyle:

1. Minimize all processed foods, as they tend to be loaded with sugar and salt.

2. Eat modest portions of beef, poultry, and pork, and at each meal, try not to eat a serving size of meat that's bigger than a deck of cards.

3. Limit sugar, particularly sugary drinks, which are the leading source of added sugar in our diets. These added sugars are linked to obesity, diabetes, elevated LDL (bad cholesterol), diminished HDL (good cholesterol), and elevated fat in the blood.

4. Eat more whole grains, nuts, fruits, vegetables, and beans. Try to make them staples of your diet. These foods have those all-powerful heart-protecting antioxidants, plus helpful fiber and healthy fats.

5. Fat consumption is not your adversary. Just try to avoid foods packed with saturated fat such as meat, cheese, and butter. Some fatty foods, like nuts, seeds, olive oil, and salmon, are packed with heart-healthy unsaturated fats. Enjoy these healthier fats in moderation.

6. It's OK to start eating eggs again. The newest evidence suggests that the intake of eggs does not impact your cholesterol levels as we once thought.

7. If you drink alcohol, limit your intake. Women should have no more than one alcoholic drink per day. Men should have no more than two alcoholic drinks per day.

8. Do 30 minutes or more of moderate-intensity (somewhat hard) physical activity on most days of the week.

CHAPTER 8

Let's Get Up and Start Moving Now!

BEFORE I INTRODUCE YOUR HIIT WORKOUTS, I'D LIKE TO ENCOURAGE YOU TO START GET-
ting up more in your daily life. Yes, that includes standing up from your chairs. If your home is your castle, its chairs have become the throne. It won't guarantee you bountiful riches, though—at least not of the good-health variety. Over the past few years, a large group of scientists have been studying what happens to our bodies when we sit too much. It is called the science of sedentary behavior. The word "sedentary" comes from the Latin word *sedere*, meaning "to sit." In the US, sedentary behavior takes up a great percentage of the waking day for many people. In fact, adults and children in the US spend the majority of their non-exercising waking day engaging in some form of sedentary behavior, such as riding in a car, working at a desk, eating a meal at a table, playing video games, working on a computer, and watching television. You will probably not be surprised to learn that a sedentary lifestyle can have hazardous health effects. Researchers increasingly believe that, as the saying goes, sitting has become the new smoking.

Findings about the harmful effects of too much sitting have their early research roots in the 1950s, when researchers observed that men who worked physically active jobs had less heart disease during middle age than men in physically inactive jobs. The researchers also observed that when physically active men *did* develop heart disease, it was less severe and later in life. Leaping forward half a century, in 2009, a large study from Canada found that there is a strong association between sitting and mortality risk from cardiovascular disease (and several other diseases, too). This study, published in *Medicine & Science in Sports & Exercise*, looked at the mortality rates of 7,278 men and 9,735 women aged eighteen to ninety years over a twelve-year period. Surprisingly, the study discovered that even if a person completes her/his 30 minutes of moderate-intensity exercise a day but remains seated during the rest of the day, she/he has an increased risk of heart disease. The bottom line: long periods of sitting during your waking day are unsafe to your health.

Why is it so unhealthy to sit for sustained periods of time on a daily basis? Scientist believe when you sit too much during your waking day, the bad cholesterol (LDL cholesterol) starts to accumulate more plaque in your arteries. Simultaneously, the good cholesterol (HDL cholesterol) decreases, making it less available for cleaning up the plaque. Once a lot of plaque builds up in your arteries, you are vulnerable to cardiovascular disease.

All of the new research on the perils of a sedentary lifestyle underscores the critical importance of getting up and moving much more throughout your waking day. To help you accomplish this, I'm going to reveal a NEW slogan and goal I'd like you to shoot for every day: "For every 30, get your 3."

Here's how it works: for every 30 minutes you sit, I want you to get at least 3 minutes of movement. Yes, more is better, but to start let's shoot for "For every 30, get your 3." I realize some jobs, due to their nature, do not allow you to take a movement break every 30 minutes. I encourage those of you in such a situation to find creative ways to achieve your movement goals over the course of your workday. However, many of you *will* be able to get up out of your chairs and move every 30 minutes without any restrictions. You get to decide how far and how fast you move—but just move. So start right now—get up and move! Go for it, and then come back to reading your book. I will do the same.

[A few minutes pass] . . . and we're back. See, didn't that feel great?

To help you get moving, here are some options for breaking up sustained sitting periods at work:

1. Standing up and walking around your work office every 30 minutes.

2. Standing up and moving every time you drink some water.

3. Walking to the farthest bathroom in your worksite facility when going to the restroom (if multiple bathrooms are available).

4. Standing and/or walking around the room when talking on the telephone.

5. Getting a standing workstation where you can intermittently stand and work on your desktop computer simultaneously.

6. Going for a walk break during every coffee or tea break.

7. Substituting sending emails to office colleagues by walking to their desks to communicate with them personally.

8. Making your next meeting a walking/talking/discussing meeting.

Of course, excessive sitting doesn't happen only at work; it's just as much of a problem once you get home. Many people spend a lot of time—perhaps too much time—watching TV, viewing movies, and/or reading books in a chair. To help counteract the effects of this, please do some of the following at home:

1. Getting up and moving during every commercial.

2. Taking a brief walk break every 30 minutes.

3. Getting on a stationary piece of cardiovascular exercise equipment, such as a treadmill or indoor cycle) and using it for several minutes after each half-hour of TV viewing or reading.

4. Standing up and moving for the opening segment of each TV show.

5. Getting up to walk around the room or house every time you read four, six, or eight pages.

TAKEAWAYS FROM THE SEDENTARY BEHAVIOR RESEARCH

Our technologically advanced society has given us the opportunity to do almost everything we need to from our chairs. While this may have some work productivity benefits, being sedentary for so long can be very damaging to your health. In addition to enjoying the many great HIIT workouts in this book, I want you to strive to fulfill your new movement slogan on a daily basis: "For every 30, get your 3." You can do it! Please be empowered and encouraged to teach it to your family and close friends as well. Remember, the ultimate power lies in the lifestyle choices you make every day. Get up, move, and enjoy!

Optimal Weight (Fat) Loss Strategies That Work!

CHAPTER 9

Successful Weight Management; "Inch by Inch, It's a Cinch"

AS YOU PROBABLY KNOW, OBESITY IS A MAJOR HEALTH ISSUE IN MANY COUNTRIES throughout the world—including our own. According to World Health Organization (WHO) data from 2017, the rate of obesity in the world has nearly tripled since 1975. Recent 2018 data from the Centers for Disease Control and Prevention indicates that more than one-third of US adults, 36.5%, are obese, a staggering statistic. As alarming as this is, contained within this list of key facts and statistics is the following statement from the WHO: "Obesity is preventable." I want you to always remember that inspiring, valuable message.

Losing weight, and maintaining the weight loss, is definitely a worldwide challenge facing millions of women and men. But it is important to emphasize that even small changes in body weight can result in consequential health benefits. Studies show that a 5% to 10% loss of initial body weight, which is very doable, is associated with meaningful improvements in cholesterol levels, blood pressure (when elevated), and in the management and prevention of type 2 diabetes. For that very reason, a target goal of many weight-loss programs is for participants to lose at least 10% of one's initial weight, and then maintain that loss for a minimum of one year. I assure you, this is a realistic and achievable goal.

Before we get started, it's probably best to get a major weight loss disclaimer out of the way: it is clear from hundreds of research articles and weight loss books that there is no *one* best approach to successful weight loss. Just as there isn't one best diet or dietary style, there isn't one best exercise program; in fact, there isn't even one best HIIT program. Indeed, in the long run, you and every other person who strives to meet weight management goals will eventually find what works best for you. However, the research does show there are some evidence-based strategies that work very well for many people, and there are some important dietary and exercise approaches that are most beneficial health-wise. These are the strategies we are going to go over in this book. Think of these approaches as some of the tools of the weight management success toolbox.

LAUNCHING "INCH BY INCH, IT'S A CINCH"

In this chapter I will go into further detail about my "Inch by inch, it's a cinch" philosophy. As I explained earlier in the book, this is the method I've used for years while working with people trying to meet their weight management, fitness, and health goals. This philosophy is actually based on the small-changes approach, a scientific approach to behavior change. The small-changes approach encourages people to make modest but progressive behavior changes to lose weight and prevent the gradual regain of weight that has been lost. It's important to note that this strategy is meant to make you think about your diet and physical well-being as part of your lifestyle. The concept isn't suggesting that little changes will have an immediately greater impact than some aggressive approaches to weight loss. Quite the contrary! But, for many people, the small-changes approach is a part of an achievable lifestyle, which is much more sustainable over the long run compared to disruptive, aggressive strategies that upend your life. This is really the key to weight loss success and weight regain prevention. *Lasting* changes in health, weight management, and fitness rarely come from quick fix approaches. Don't allow yourself to become enticed—or, rather, hoodwinked—by the slick advertising and marketing of some rapid weight loss product or program. With any program you consider, see if there is evidence supporting the program beyond the testimonials you hear or read in the advertising.

That said, it is just fine if you want to overhaul some aspects of your lifestyle. Most of us are self-improving regularly, whether we realize it or not, and sometimes changes we make definitely feel like a personal lifestyle overhaul. Fundamentally, however, I've found the "Inch by inch, it's a cinch" philosophy to be the best way to achieve your long-lasting behavior change goals. As you progress, I encourage you to welcome new healthy habits into your lifestyle.

IS THERE ANY SCIENCE TO USING A SMALL-CHANGES APPROACH?

Yes—and a lot of it! In 2009, a seventeen-member task force from the American Society for Nutrition, the Institute of Food Technologists, and the International Food Information Council was established to evaluate the efficacy of small-changes obesity intervention for a large part of the overweight/obese population. According to results published by this task force in the *American Journal of Clinical Nutrition*, this approach to combating obesity is beneficial for the following reasons:

1. **SMALL, REALISTIC CHANGES ARE EASIER TO ACHIEVE AND MAINTAIN THAN LARGE ONES.** The committee drew on years of research and observation when it found that major behavioral and lifestyle changes are quite difficult to attain. Small changes such as two thousand more steps of walking a day (which requires about 100 extra calories of energy expenditure) and simple food substitutions (such as replacing a twelve-ounce regular soda with a diet soda, saving 150 kilocalories) are doable and maintainable.

2. **SMALL CHANGES CAN HAVE AN IMPORTANT IMPACT ON BODY WEIGHT REGULATION.** Most people in the US steadily gain weight over time, because we increase the discrepancy between energy intake (food consumption) and energy output (exercise and physical activity). This discrepancy is sometimes referred to as an energy gap, and it is estimated to be up to 100 calories (or more) each day for the average American, leading people to become overweight and obese over time if it's not derailed somewhere along the way.

3. **SMALL, SUCCESSFUL LIFESTYLE CHANGES LEAD TO AN INCREASE IN POSITIVE SELF-EFFICACY.** Self-efficacy is your impression about your ability to perform in a certain manner. Positive self-efficacy when it comes to weight management suggests that as you make small lifestyle changes and achieve certain weight loss goals, you become empowered, skilled, confident, and motivated to stay on course with your goals. In fact, this increased self-confidence in yourself may inspire you to tackle even greater weight loss goals than you originally thought were possible. It's a praiseworthy cycle: positive outcomes lead to self-confidence and self-efficacy, encouraging you to make even higher gains. What could

be more empowering? Little by little, step-by-step, inch by inch, you become more and more confident in yourself and what you can achieve—at any age or stage in your life!

Is the small-changes approach right for you? Reflect for a moment. Trying to get fit or lose weight often feels overwhelming, like being lost in a giant obstacle course. This is particularly true if you have been sedentary for a long time. A big part of the problem is that many weight management programs tend to create an all-or-nothing approach, which often leads to failure and dropping out. I advise you to stay away from those programs. The small-changes approach surely deserves your genuine attention. Stay patient and goal-focused as you progress with your personal lifestyle modifications and changes. Eventually you will come to agree with me: "Inch by inch, it's a cinch."

CHAPTER 10

Lessons from *The Biggest Loser*

YOU ARE PROBABLY FAMILIAR WITH THE POPULAR TELEVISION COMPETITION SHOW *The Biggest Loser,* but if you're not, here's a quick summary: during the course of a season, participants (who are overweight or obese) battle it out to see who can lose the most amount of weight through diet and exercise. By the end of the competition, the contestants have lost dozens of pounds. As you can imagine, losing so much weight over such a short period of time requires some pretty drastic dieting and exercising measures. You might say the show's philosophy is the opposite of inch-by-inch, it's a cinch.

Whatever you think of the show—and it has generated no small amount of controversy—it has been valuable to researchers because the contestants are, essentially, subjects of a real-life experiment. Studying them could, in fact, answer this important question: do people who undertake extreme weight loss stay healthy and fit after the show is over (that is, long term)?

Well, let's look at the research to find out. In 2016, a study was published in the journal Obesity summarizing the long-term weight loss results of several contestants on the 2009 *Biggest Loser* season. The study followed fourteen contestants (six men and eight women) from the season for six years, finding that the majority had regained a substantial amount of weight. The study findings explain what happened, so we will explore them in greater detail in the next section.

RESTING METABOLIC RATE CHANGES WITH WEIGHT LOSS

First, though, let's talk briefly about your body's energy balance. Your total daily energy expenditure consists of three main categories: the resting metabolic rate (RMR), the energy needed to stay alive; the thermic effect of food (TEF), the energy required for the digestion, absorption, transport, and storage of all the foods you eat; and the activity energy expenditure (AEE), the energy the body utilizes during exercise and spontaneous physical movement (such as shopping, moving, doing daily chores, and fidgeting). Your RMR is the largest portion of the body's energy expenditure, comprising an enormous 60–70% of your daily total energy expenditure (TEE). You have a very complex body, with trillions of cells, and it requires a lot of energy to stay alive.

Here's how this is related to *The Biggest Loser*. The 2016 study discovered that rapid, severe weight loss causes a massive slowdown in the body's RMR. In science, this process is referred to as a "metabolic adaptation." As the researchers of the study explain, metabolic adaptation occurs when the body tries to counteract such drastic weight loss. In other words, the body slows down its RMR in hopes of *gaining back* the lost weight. For the Obesity study, researchers measured contestants' RMR at the beginning of the 2009 *Biggest Loser* season, at the end of the 30-week competition, and six years after that. (See Table 1 for details from the assessment.)

Table 1. Body Composition & Energy Expenditure Comparisons

VARIABLE	PRE-CONTEST	30 WEEKS	6 YEARS AFTER
Body Weight (lbs.)	328	200	290
Body Fat (%)	49.3	28.1	44.7
Muscle Mass (lbs.)	166	142	155
Fat Mass (lbs.)	162	58	135
RMR (calories/day)	2607	1,996	1,903
TEE (calories/day)	3,804	3,002	3,429

Values are averages of the 6 men and 8 women in the *Biggest Loser* contest before the start of the contest (Pre-Contest), immediately after the contest (30 weeks), and 6 years after the contest. Source: Fothergill et al., 2016.

On average, the fourteen contestants each lost 128 pounds in the 30-week weight loss competition. At the six-year follow-up, researchers found, the contestants had gained back an average of 90 pounds The contestants lost 24 pounds of muscle during the vigorous 30-week exercise program, but gained back 13 pounds of muscle six years after the contest. Likewise, the contestants lost an average of 104 pounds of fat in the 30-week contest, but gained back 77 pounds of fat by the six-year assessment. Perhaps the most startling result, and one that helps explain the contestants' weight *regain*, has to do with their RMR measurements.

At the completion of the 30-week contest, the average measured RMR of each contestant was 611 calories lower than at the start of it. Surprisingly, at the six-year follow-up, each contestant's RMR was on average 93 calories LOWER than after the 30-week exercise/nutrition intervention. Thus, from the pre-contest time to the six-year follow-up, each contestant's RMR was suppressed by an average of 704 calories. In other words, their bodies were trying hard to gain back the lost weight by severely slowing down their RMR. This is gripping—and surprising to learn.

DID THE CONTESTANTS' RAPID WEIGHT LOSS CAUSE THEIR WEIGHT REGAIN?

In a word: yes. Many weight management professionals maintain that *The Biggest Loser* participants' extreme, rapid loss experience directly contributed to their subsequent weight regain. With the dramatic slowing of their RMR, their bodies were expending fewer calories on a daily basis, and they gained back a substantial amount of weight. Weight loss and fitness professionals, myself included, believe it is unhealthy to lose massive amounts of weight so quickly, especially through the extreme fitness regimens contestants endure in the show, such as 7 hours of exercise a day. This is one of the reasons I am such a strong champion for the "Inch by inch, it's a cinch" philosophy in fitness and weight management. It allows for the body to gradually adjust to the small changes in body weight that occur over a period of time. Numerous studies have shown small progressive changes are quite doable and sustainable over the long run.

IS IT TRUE THAT DIETING-ONLY PROGRAMS CAN ACTUALLY PROMOTE GAIN WEIGHT?

As the name implies, diet-only weight-loss programs do not include any type of exercise. To figure out how this approach fares, let's look to the science. In a 2012 study published in the *International Journal of Obesity*, researchers collected and reported on weight changes among 4,129 individual twins at sixteen-, seventeen-, eighteen-, and twenty-five-year increments after the start of the study. In the report, the researchers confirmed that a dieting-only weight-loss program may lead to the *opposite* of the desired weight loss outcome. The authors hypothesize that restrictive dieting may lead some people to become preoccupied with food and trigger overeating. In addition, the researchers found that the suppression of the RMR and loss of muscle mass may spur post-dieting weight-rebound—the same conclusion of the study of *The Biggest Loser* contestants. As we discussed, a post-dieting weight rebound appears to be a response by the body, which is reacting defensively to the weight loss. These reactions may be part psychological and part physiological, but the fact is that this rebounding leads to regaining lost weight. In some cases, people will actually wind up weighing *more* than when they originally started their diet. All of which is to say: yes, it appears that dieting-only weight-loss programs can indeed lead to weight gain. The great news is that there are several ways to combat this weight regain phenomenon, and we will cover them thoroughly in the next chapter, Secrets from Real-Life Biggest Losers.

CHAPTER 11

Secrets from Real-Life Biggest Losers

GIVEN HOW MUCH CONSUMER ADVERTISING IS DOMINATED BY DIET BOOKS AND WEIGHT- loss products and programs touting sketchy, quick-fix solutions, one could be forgiven for despairing when it comes to viable long-term weight-loss programs that actually work. Despair not, however; the truth is, there *are* real-life biggest losers who have successfully maintained long-term weight loss. To learn what these real-life biggest losers have been doing right, we will turn our attention to the National Weight Control Registry (NWCR), an archive of thousands of women and men who have lost 30 pounds or more, and kept it off.

In this chapter we will analyze the NWCR data to figure out what *really* worked for those who have attained successful long-term weight loss and prevented weight regain. My hope is that their experiences and lessons can serve as insightful guideposts for you on your own journey.

INTRODUCING THE NATIONAL WEIGHT CONTROL REGISTRY

The NWCR was established by doctors Jim Hill and Rena Wing in 1994. The registry was developed for the express purpose of categorizing and examining the behavior of individuals who have succeeded at long-term weight loss. All of the ten thousand plus members currently in the registry are at least eighteen years or older, have lost at least 30 pounds, and have maintained this weight loss for at least one year. Eighty percent of the people in the registry are women, and 20% are men. The average woman in the registry is forty-five years old and currently weighs 145 pounds, while the average man in it is forty-nine and currently weighs 190 pounds. NWCR volunteers (there is no compensation for participating) are recruited using national and local television, radio, magazine, and newspaper advertisements. Each new member first calls a toll-free number or completes a web application to determine his or her eligibility for the NWCR, and then (if eligible to join) they are sent a consent form and detailed questionnaire packet that includes questions about the following: lifetime maximum weight (and dates at this weight), current weight, education, ethnicity, age, gender, exercise habits, and methods of weight loss used. All registry members are tracked annually to determine any weight changes that have occurred as well as associated weight-related behavior modifications, if any.

Most NWCR members have lost an average of 66 pounds and kept this weight off for 5.5 years. (Praise where praise is due—that is exceedingly impressive!) The number of pounds lost ranges from 30 to 300 pounds, and the duration of sustained weight loss ranges from one year to sixty-six years. Some of the registry members lost their weight rapidly, while others lost it rather slowly, over a period up to fourteen years. Remarkably, 45% of registry participants lost the weight on their own, while the other 55% lost weight with the help of some type of program such as a commercial diet program, or with the guidance of a physician or nutritionist. Ninety-eight percent of the registry members report they modified their food intake in some way to lose weight, and 94% increased their physical activity, with the most frequently reported form of activity being walking. Most of the registry members watch fewer than 10 hours of television per week. This tells us they are definitely combatting the challenges of sedentary behavior.

WHAT STRATEGIES HAVE WORKED FOR THESE LONG-TERM WEIGHT-LOSS WINNERS?

If we dig into the data, we can uncover the four main strategies NWCR members rely on for successful weight loss maintenance:

1. Doing high levels of physical activity

2. Consuming a lower-calorie diet

3. Weighing themselves frequently (i.e., monitoring their weight)

4. Eating breakfast, typically cereal (low-fat and low-sugar breakfast foods) and fruit, every day

Additionally, there are certain personality traits that successful weight loss "losers" have in common, most notably a heightened sense of vigilance about maintaining their weight loss. For instance, survey reports of this population reveal that successful weight loss maintainers *continue to act like recently successful weight-loss losers* for many years after their weight loss. In other words, they are "laser focused" when it comes to maintaining their lighter weight, and keep up this laser focus day after day. Seventy-five percent of NWCR members weigh themselves at least once a week, and 44% of registry members weigh themselves daily, further demonstrating the importance of their regular body monitoring.

HOW MUCH PHYSICAL ACTIVITY DO REGISTRY MEMBERS GET?

Both men and women on the registry get a lot of physical activity each week, a fact that is probably unsurprising. Both sexes average up to 1 hour each day of physical activity at a somewhat hard intensity. That is like taking two brisk 30-minute walks a day: one in the morning and one in the afternoon. If we use the talk test as a guide, when you are working at a somewhat hard intensity you can exercise and carry on a conversation with a little bit of difficulty.

Seventy-six percent of members report that walking is their main form of physical activity. Other physical activities reported by men and women in the registry include resistance training, cycling, and other aerobic activities. Previous research on this population shows that as registry members decrease their physical activity, they have a tendency to regain some weight. So, regular exercise surely plays a key role in the prevention of weight regain for this population.

WHAT HAPPENS TO NWCR REGISTRY MEMBERS WHO REGAIN WEIGHT?

Researchers examined registry members who regained >5 pounds after one year of weight loss success to determine what predictors might indicate a member's likelihood of weight regain. They found that those who regain weight tend to periodically lose control of their eating. Also, those with higher levels of depression showed greater odds for regaining weight. It also appears that an increase in the percentage of calories from fat in a member's diet is associated with some weight regain.

However, perhaps the most important (if not most inspiring) finding is that members who were successful at maintaining their weight loss for two or more years had *significantly greater chances of keeping weight off throughout the subsequent years*. If women and men can succeed at maintaining their weight loss for two years, they can reduce their risk of subsequent weight regain by nearly 50%. Although this phenomenon is not fully understood, one explanation is that people who maintain their weight for at least two years have developed successful long-term coping skills that further equip them to manage their weight loss.

WHAT SPARKS MOST PEOPLE IN THE NWCR TO INITIALLY START THEIR WEIGHT LOSS PLAN?

It appears that the majority (83%) of the men and women in the NWCR have some type of prompt or trigger that sets off their weight loss initiative. The three most common prompts for weight loss and continued maintenance include medical conditions (23%), reaching an all-time high in body weight (21.3%), and observing oneself in a mirror or a picture (12.7%). Medical reasons were generally described as conditions that would lead to a heart attack if nothing were done. The next two motivators that follow the top three include wanting to live a longer life and/or having more time to spend with loved ones. In my view, it's interesting that simply getting a slimmer body isn't what motivates the majority of registry members.

Quite a few members acknowledge that they had previously made several failed attempts to lose weight before finding what really works for them. Many can attest that they are quite familiar with "yo-yo" dieting (losing and regaining weight in a cyclical manner). This is important for everyone starting a fitness, health, and/or weight-loss program to know: there are a lot of ups and downs, just like a roller coaster, before you really find what works best for you when it comes to exercise and weight management. The majority of the NWCR registry members maintained their motivation during these trying times and finally succeeded. You will too!

WHAT DO NWCR MEMBERS' DIETS HAVE IN COMMON?

We can learn a lot from the commonalities between NWCR members, especially when it comes to diet. To start, members appeared to share an appreciation for consistency and a determination to stick with a dietary regimen. Fifty-nine percent of members said their eating habits were the same on weekends (and holidays) and weekdays, while 39% of participants noted they followed stricter diets during the week as compared to the weekend. This is an important concept to discuss. I have worked with many people who have a tendency to eat and drink heavily on the weekends. It is important to realize weekends can be unpredictable, but to always focus on your short- and long-term dietary goals, as these NWCR members demonstrate. Notably, NWCR members who are more consistent with their diets during the week and weekend are 1.5 times more likely to maintain weight loss during the next year. This outcome seems to be validated by research. In a 2005 study published in the *American Journal of Clinical Nutrition*, researchers assert that allowing for "too much flexibility" in dietary behaviors may expose a person to high-risk situations, creating more opportunity to lose control and eat too much. So, during weekends, when you may enjoy special outings with your family, friends, and colleagues, please be aware of placing yourself in a tempting situation where you may overindulge. Enjoy, but perhaps remind yourself to use moderation.

PRACTICAL ADVICE FROM REAL-LIFE BIGGEST LOSERS

To help you lose weight and achieve long-term weight control, here's a summary of the most important lessons we can draw from the National Weight Control Registry's ten thousand plus real-life biggest losers.

1. No two people lost weight in exactly the same way in the registry. Accordingly, you must find what works best for you. In many ways, this gives you the permission to explore different kinds of weight loss options; just know that there is a weight management plan, strategy, or program out there that will work for you, even if it takes some time to find it.

2. All of the members on the registry have a sincere motivation for achieving their goals, whether it is a medical scare, an all-time high weight, or just wanting to spend more time with family and friends. Clearly, there are different factors that motivate people to be successful in weight management.

3. Whether they came to it on their own, or from joining a weight loss group or program, all members of the registry modified their diet in a way to take in fewer calories. How do you plan to modify your diet? What steps do you plan to take? If you're not sure, remember

that this book includes a special chapter with one hundred ways to reduce calories in your daily life. Please take advantage of many of these fabulous ideas—they are my gift to you.

4. The majority of members of the registry complete up to 1 hour of somewhat hard intensity exercise on most days of the week. That is the equivalent of a 30-minute brisk walk in the morning and one in the afternoon.

5. Regardless of how much time they spend exercising, most members do the same physical activity: walking briskly. Crucially, they keep up this exercise regime even after their weight loss, a strategy that definitely helps prevent weight regain.

6. A great majority of the members on the registry eat a healthy breakfast, typically cereal (low-fat and low-sugar breakfast foods) and fruit. Talk about giving yourself a healthy start!

7. Registry members weigh themselves frequently. Some check their weight daily, with most of them checking their weight at least once per week. What is best for you? Once a week? Daily? Decide and then start monitoring your weight.

8. Weight loss success is likelier to occur among members who don't let their dietary habits stray on the weekend. They are careful not to get out of control with their weekend food choices at parties, social events, and family outings. Plan ahead so you don't get caught off guard at these social occasions.

9. Most of the members on the registry have developed effective coping mechanisms to deal with any depression they may experience in their daily life. Depression is a widespread illness that affects millions of adults in the United States every year, but the good news is that it can be treated. If you believe you are depressed, getting help is the best thing you can do for yourself. Please note that depression is often associated with weight gain.

10. It's not uncommon for NWCR members to experience the cycle of yo-yo dieting (the seesawing of weight loss and weight regain) on their road to successful weight management.

Many NWCR members know what it is like to fail multiple times with dietary approaches. Weight management changes can be challenging for all of us. Have a positive attitude and be encouraged to reach out to your health practitioner, a certified personal trainer, or a registered dietician for guidance. Like the many thousands of people on the NWCR, you too can be healthy and happy.

11. Many members of the registry have effective self-monitoring techniques. Besides weighing themselves often, many keep dietary and exercise journals. This may be very helpful for tracking your own journey.

12. Members get back on track if they see they are sliding off their program. In other words, they do not let a small lapse turn into a big relapse. Likewise, I always encourage the people I work with to keep a laser focus on their goals. If they get off track, they should use the same laser focus to get back on their journey.

13. Members keep their emotions from affecting their diet and exercise. When faced with emotional challenges, they avoid using food as an escape.

14. The majority of the NWCR members watch less than 10 hours of TV per week, a major victory in the battle to combat sedentary behavior. I encourage you to do the same.

15. NWCR members have developed an incredible vigilance when it comes to sticking with their exercise and dietary program. How inspiring. You can do this too!

16. Members who successfully maintain their weight loss for over two years significantly increase their odds for continued long-term success.

The most important message to take from these ten thousand plus real-life biggest losers is that losing weight and getting fit is really doable—for anyone. Learn from their success strategies and let their successes embolden you. Now is YOUR time to succeed. You can do it! Remember, "Inch by inch, it's a cinch!"

CHAPTER 12

What's the Healthiest Diet for Me?

YOU KNOW FROM THE PREVIOUS CHAPTER THAT THERE IS NO ONE DIETARY APPROACH that works best. The members of the National Weight Control Registry each established their own dietary plans (many with guidance from a program or health practitioner) and exercise routines to stay fit. So, the concept of one "best" diet has to be overruled. That said, some diets are definitely healthier than others! (A diet centered around fried food obviously isn't as healthy as one centered around vegetables and healthy fats.)

When it comes to healthy diets, a Mediterranean-type diet is worth your full attention. The traditional Mediterranean diet is rich in intake of fresh fruits, vegetables, legumes, nuts, fish, olive oil, and whole grains. It encourages eaters to minimize their intake of saturated fats, processed meat, added sugar, and refined grains. The diet is well-known for supporting a moderate intake of alcohol, specifically wine, with meals. The Mediterranean diet is linked to several major health benefits including reduced cancer risk, enhanced cardioprotection, a decrease in nervous disorders, and an overall reduction in mortality.

A study published in the *British Medical Journal* in 2014, offers some promising indications that the Mediterranean diet may lead to a longer life. This research examined records from 4,676 healthy middle-aged female nurses (average age = fifty-nine years, ranging between forty-two and seventy) who were involved in the Nurses' Health Study, an ongoing study tracking the health of more than 120,000 US nurses since 1976. Every other year the participants in the Nurses' Health Study complete questionnaires on health information, lifestyle activities, and diagnoses of diseases. And, every four years since 1984, researchers ask study participants to complete food intake questionnaires, to fully identify what they were eating on a daily basis. As you can imagine, this has resulted in a large, ongoing investigation with lots of useful data for researchers. Let's now shift gears briefly and discuss telomeres.

WHAT ARE TELOMERES?

The word "telomeres" comes from the Greek words *telos* ("end") and *meros* ("part"). Accordingly, telomeres are the end parts or caps at the end of each strand of DNA. They protect our chromosomes and are like the plastic tips at the end of shoelaces or the eraser on the tip of a pencil. Your chromosomes are thread-like structures that house your DNA molecules. As for DNA, it contains the biological instructions for the development and functioning of all known living organisms. Telomeres are vital because they keep your chromosomes from unraveling (remember, they are the end parts). However, it's possible for your telomeres to be damaged by villain molecules.

This is a lot to take in, but bear with me! Sometimes, when your cells give off reactions, they make these molecules that are very harmful. These molecules are known as free radicals, and they are so harmful because they're missing an electron, a vital component of molecular structure. Free radicals are very unstable in their new form, and to become stable they must find another electron. This means they will go anywhere in the cell to steal an electron—to your DNA, other proteins, or other parts of a cell. This unhealthy condition, during which free radicals steal other electrons, is called "oxidative stress." Scientists now know these free radicals like to eat away at our telomeres. This is very damaging, and reduces the strength and protective effectiveness of your telomeres. Once these dangerous free radical molecules build up in your cells, their cell damage is linked to aging and age-related diseases.

Fortunately, there is a happy ending to this somber story, so please keep reading. The 2014 *British Medical Journal* study confirmed what other researchers have shown: that telomere length is considered a biomarker of aging. In other words, a person with shorter telomeres may have a decreased life expectancy and increased susceptibility to chronic diseases. A person with lengthier telomeres is likely to have a longer life expectancy with fewer health consequences. Many scientists now also believe the length of someone's telomeres is closely associated with the person's dietary patterns and lifestyle practices.

That's the great news: *you can actively contribute to the health of your telomeres through your own choices.* This is where the Mediterranean diet comes in. This type of diet helps the body produce powerful molecules that literally neutralize those dangerous free radical molecules. Yes, at the cellular level, we have some really neat superhero molecules—we call them "antioxidants." They don't wear a cape, but these are superheroes that deactivate free radicals, ensuring these bad molecules can no longer cause harm. I know this reads like a story in a comic book, but it's real science! The researchers in the *British Medical Journal study* explain that adherence to the Mediterranean diet is associated with making more of these specialized antioxidants. This same research team examined the relationship between higher adherence to the Mediterranean diet and telomere length in the group of US women who participated in the Nurses' Health study. The results are in the next section.

DOES A MEDITERRANEAN DIET LEAD TO LONGER TELOMERES?

First and foremost, it's a fact that telomeres shorten with age, even in healthy people. Accordingly, the scientists in the Nurses' Health study noted that the younger women had longer telomeres than the older women. Alas, shorter telomeres are also related to aging and age-related diseases such as liver disease, atherosclerosis, and certain cancers. But the great news from this *British Medical Journal* study is that the results indicate that those participants who followed a Mediterranean diet had longer telomeres. These results support the Mediterranean diet's role in promoting health and a person's lifespan. In essence, aspects of the Mediterranean diet enhance your body's ability to prevent or delay heart disease, stroke, and type 2 diabetes.

WHAT ARE THE MECHANISMS OF THE MEDITERRANEAN DIET THAT PROMOTE LONGEVITY?

Obviously, the big question arising from this study is: what is it about the Mediterranean diet that promotes longevity? The researchers believe that the anti-aging effects of the diet come from the nutrient-rich foods that are typically part of it. According to the researchers, it's unlikely that one single food is responsible for the diet's health benefits; rather, the benefits likely come from eating multiple staples of the diet in combination.

ARE THERE ANY LIMITATIONS OF THIS STUDY?

The researchers note that the Nurses' Health Study population primarily includes women of European lineage. Telomere length may differ among people of different genders and ethnicities, so the results of this study cannot be generalized to all people in the world (at least at this time). As a result, I will make the typical scientist's disclaimer: more research is needed to confirm these same results within other ethnic populations.

HOW DOES PHYSICAL ACTIVITY EFFECT TELOMERE LENGTH?

One of the first studies to measure telomere length and physical activity was published in *PLOS ONE* in 2011. In the study, researchers investigated the effect of low fitness, moderate fitness, and high fitness levels and telomere length in 944 male and female patients with coronary heart disease. The researchers showed that people with a low fitness level had 94% greater odds of having short telomere length as compared to those with a high fitness level, leading the researchers to conclude that there is a clear, direct linkage between longer telomere length and higher cardiorespiratory fitness level. The scientists propose that cardiorespiratory exercise may activate regulatory proteins that control telomere length; while they don't know for certain, we will surely learn more about this in the next few years. Whatever the specific cause, the take-home message is clear: high levels of aerobic fitness are associated with longer, protective telomeres. One of the greatest benefits of HIIT workouts is the positive effect they have on developing your aerobic fitness—and by extension, your telomeres. I hope it's gratifying to know that HIIT workouts are some of the most beneficial types of exercise you can do.

LET'S TALK ABOUT INFLAMMATION

The 2014 study in the *British Medical Journal* determined that the Mediterranean diet also helps to control chronic inflammation. Inflammation is a self-protection and healing response by the body to remove harmful stimuli, irritants, pathogens, and/or damaged cells. Inflammation comes in two major categories: acute, which occurs for a short period of time, and chronic, which can last for months or years. In most instances, inflammation is a brief response to an incident, such as spraining an ankle. Symptoms of inflammation include swelling, redness, pain, and impaired movement or function. While uncomfortable, inflammation is how the body protects and heals itself. With acute inflammation, the body targets the damaged area and sends specialized healing cells to the area to promote healing. This kind of inflammation ends as healing proceeds.

Chronic inflammation is the threatening kind of inflammation. Whenever you hear doctors or scientists speaking to the media about the hazards of inflammation, it's chronic inflammation they're talking about. With chronic inflammation, the body's immune system attacks healthy cells, mistaking them for harmful cells. So, whenever you hear the words chronic inflammation, know that it means some part of the immune system is trying to heal an area of the body, but the healing proteins accidently attack healthy cells instead. For instance, rheumatoid arthritis is an example of chronic inflammation. Rheumatoid arthritis affects the lining of your joints, causing a painful swelling that continually persists, leading to bone and joint damage.

Perhaps unsurprisingly, obesity is also associated with chronic inflammation. Some researchers believe that overeating increases the body's immune response, thus prompting an excess of inflammatory molecules in the blood. This increased immune response becomes chronic inflammation, which in turn increases a person's odds of developing chronic diseases such as type 2 diabetes and cardiovascular disease.

SHOULD YOU CHOOSE THE MEDITERRANEAN DIET?

The diet you choose is ultimately up to you. But our understanding of telomeres and how a Mediterranean diet may positively influence them—thus leading to a longer, healthier life—is encouraging. It's also reassuring to read about the positive effects aerobic exercise has on telomere length, because you are going to get a lot of great HIIT workout ideas from this book. However, choosing your diet is a very personal decision. Remember the ten thousand plus members of the National Weight Control Registry; of this large group, no two people are on precisely the same diet. So the choice is yours. As I've noted several times in this book, *you are in control of your life and have the power to make the best choices for you.*

CHAPTER 13

Low-Carbohydrate versus Low-Fat Diets: What Is the Verdict?

WITHIN THE LAST TWO DECADES THERE HAVE BEEN A NUMBER OF STUDIES ATTEMPTING TO determine what's better for weight loss: a low-carbohydrate diet or a low-fat one. Indeed, we have all witnessed the low-carbohydrate versus low-fat advertisements and marketing campaigns in the media.

Before we dig into this topic, a few caveats are in order. Recall, as we discussed in the previous chapter, that of the ten thousand plus members of the National Weight Control Registry, all whom have lost at least 30 pounds and maintained this weight loss for at least a year, no two people are on the exact same diet, and also that new research suggests the Mediterranean diet might be the best eating approach when it comes to health benefits and quality of life.

That said, the low-carbohydrate versus low-fat question is unavoidable and divisive, so it is important to discuss this prominent topic in weight management. Indeed, you may decide to try both of these approaches in your journey to discover the eating style that works best for you. With that in mind let's discuss both dietary approaches, look at some of the research and then come up with a verdict.

THE CASE FOR LOW-CARBOHYDRATE DIETS

Low-carbohydrate diets revolve around the hormone insulin, a fat-producing hormone that can convert blood sugar to stored fat. When you eat foods with carbohydrates, your insulin levels become elevated. In fact, in professional weight management circles, there is a carbohydrate-insulin model of obesity, which theorizes that diets high in carbohydrates are particularly fattening due to their propensity to elevate insulin levels. Therefore, advocates of a low-carbohydrate diet believe carbohydrates are the cause of the obesity epidemic because they increase insulin in your circulating blood. The rise in insulin is the body's way of sending blood sugar (in the form of glucose) to the brain, liver, and muscles for energy, with unused glucose being stored as fat. Low-carbohydrate diet advocates claim that by limiting the intake of carbohydrates, you can avoid a rapid rise in blood sugar and thus insulin, which leads to less sugar being stored as fat.

However, some health professionals argue that rapid weight loss in low-carbohydrate diets actually comes from a striking loss of water weight. This occurs for two reasons:

1. The body stores about three parts water to every one part carbohydrate. Therefore, substantially reducing carbohydrates will dramatically lower your water (not fat) weight.

2. Low-carbohydrate diets allow for a high intake of fats as well as an increase in protein intake. By eating more proteins, the body's protein metabolism is enhanced, which requires the use of extra energy for digestion and extra water for elimination of its byproducts. Both of these processes promote weight loss.

In addition, some researchers propose people on a low-carbohydrate dietary plan are essentially eating fewer total calories. There is evidence this is correct in many cases. For instance, it has been shown that eating extra protein actually helps curb your appetite, assisting you in your goal to eat less.

THE CASE FOR LOW-FAT DIETS

Low-fat diets have been around for a long time. Fats supply energy and essential fatty acids that stimulate absorption of the fat-soluble vitamins A, D, E, and K. However, high levels of saturated fat in the diet are linked to a greater risk for heart disease and certain cancers. Thus, the goal of a low-fat diet is to target the undesirable saturated fats. Since fat, whether from plant or animal sources, has twice the number of calories as an equal amount of carbohydrate or protein, low-fat diet advocates recommend eating less fat. Fewer calories = weight loss.

Not all fats are the same. Canola and olive oils have monounsaturated fats, and most high-fat fish, vegetable oils, and nuts, are good sources of polyunsaturated fats. Both monounsaturated and polyunsaturated fats reduce blood cholesterol when they replace saturated fats in the diet. The fats in most fish are low in saturated fatty acids but contain a certain type of polyunsaturated fatty acid, known as "omega-3 fatty acids," that are associated with a decreased risk for heart disease in some people.

As a result, advocates of low-fat diets suggest mildly reducing monounsaturated and polyunsaturated (healthy) fats and dramatically lowering your intake of saturated fats. Partially hydrogenated vegetable oils, such as those used in many margarines and shortenings, contain a particular form of unsaturated fat known as "trans-fatty acids." Trans-fatty acids may raise blood cholesterol levels, thus risking heart disease. Low-fat advocates recommend eating foods with fewer trans-fatty acids as well.

WHAT DOES THE SCIENCE SHOW?
WHICH DIET IS BETTER FOR WEIGHT LOSS?

The question of whether low-carbohydrate diets or low-fat diets are superior for weight loss is a very controversial question. In 2015 and 2016, a research team from the National Institute of Diabetes and Digestive and Kidney Diseases investigated this very question in two different studies. In the highly controlled 2015 study, published in the journal *Cell Metabolism*, obese participants lived in a clinical laboratory setting for two 2-week trials. The researchers found that when obese adults ate strictly controlled diets, restricting dietary fat led to body fat loss at a rate of 68% higher than cutting the same number of carbohydrate calories. There was some good news for the reduced-carb diet, though. The low-carbohydrate diet was particularly effective at lowering insulin secretion and increasing fat burning, resulting in meaningful body fat loss. However, study participants lost more body fat during the fat-restricted diet. In the 2016 study, published in the *American Journal of Clinical Nutrition,* the results were very similar. The caveat is that the results from both studies were obtained by following dieters for a short period of time (up to 4 weeks) in a highly contained experimental environment where every morsel of food eaten was closely monitored and controlled—not exactly a simulation of real life. That said, since both dietary approaches showed positive results, the researchers suggest that the best diet may be whatever a person can stick to.

Be that as it may, let's look at just a little more research in the next section to come up with our final verdict on this debate.

THE VERDICT: LOW-FAT OR LOW-CARBOHYDRATE?

Many respected scholars argue that weight loss is more a function of consuming fewer calories, regardless of the type of food (fat, carbohydrate, protein). These same weight loss scholars recommend finding the diet that works best for you and sticking with it. Sounds a lot like the suggestions that came from studying the ten thousand plus members of the National Weight Control Registry, no? The major take-away from these highly controlled studies is that there are positive attributes to both a low-carbohydrate and low-fat dietary approach to weight loss. They both work for weight management.

In the interest of providing additional perspectives on this debate, I defer to two very reputable sources. The first source is a two-year study published in the *New England Journal of Medicine* that compared low-fat, low-carbohydrate, and the Mediterranean diets. This study found that after two years the Mediterranean and low-carbohydrate diets resulted in slightly more weight loss than the low-fat diet. Notably, there was no significant weight loss difference between the Mediterranean and the low-carbohydrate diets. In their discussion of their findings, the researchers suggested that healthcare providers should be open and willing to try all three approaches with clients to find the right diet for each individual person.

My second source is a 2014 combined position stand taken by the American Heart Association, the Obesity Society, and the American College of Cardiology and published in the journal *Circulation*. Their message was clear: Select a diet that is either low in fat, low in carbohydrates, or low in calories in order to create an energy deficit for weight loss goals.

As you've probably realized, both of these sources found precisely what we learned from the ten thousand plus members of the National Weight Control Registry. The final verdict on this longstanding dietary debate: permit yourself to try and find the right eating lifestyle that works best for you. There is a plan that will work best for YOU.

CHAPTER 14

The Stress-Cortisol-Obesity Connection

IN MANY DIFFERENT SOCIETIES, STRESS IS COMMONLY ASSOCIATED WITH NEGATIVE SITUA-
tions and settings. Yet a stress-free life may also be harmful, because it may cause an individual
to lose her or his ability to react to the different challenges of life. Every person has an optimal
positive stress level, a term referred to as "eustress," as opposed to stress that is harmful, sometimes referred to as "distress." More recent research has shown that continuing stress is highly
associated with the accumulation of abdominal fat. That's why we are going to discuss it in this
chapter and present productive ways to manage it.

WHAT IS THE EFFECT OF STRESS ON THE BODY?

People can react to a stressor in different ways. How you react to the stressor depends on if you
perceive the stress as positive, harmful, threatening, worrisome, or spurring a loss of control.
And, if the stressor's effect on you is prolonged, you may come to feel defeated, a state often
referred to as being chronically stressed. Chronic stressors are the same stressors a person deals
with week after week, month after month. Becoming, say, the caregiver for a chronically ill
family member is the type of event that might cause someone to become chronically stressed.
Chronic stress, which varies from person to person, can also occur when everyday stressors are
poorly managed or ignored and become persistent.

Chronic stress activates an area in the brain known as the hypothalamus. When this happens, hormonal signals flow from your brain, resulting in the release of cortisol, a hormone that

regulates metabolism and the body's immune responses. It has an important role in helping the body respond to stress. Cortisol is released from an area on top of each kidney known as the adrenal cortex, and it is capable of tapping into the body's fat stores and relocating fat from one location to another. Usually, cortisol helps deliver fat to tissues that need it, such as working muscle. Under chronic stressful conditions, however, cortisol may relocate fat to fat-pad sites deep in the abdomen. These are deep fat areas scientists call "central fat"; to nonscientists, they are simply the place for belly fat. When you are chronically stressed, the brain is actually trying to protect the body by putting fat in the trunk region of your body, to safeguard many of your vital organs (and some bodily systems like your heart and blood vessels). That's right; your brain is smart enough to detect your distress calls and take actions to protect your vital organs.

Researchers have discovered that the fat cells located in the deeper layers of fat in the abdominal area have more cortisol receptors compared to the fat cells underneath your skin. This makes it very easy for the body to deposit fat in the trunk area, particularly during periods of chronic stress. You see, persistent stress in your life can very well lead to unwanted belly fat. If you have experienced chronic stress, you may have observed this phenomenon. Now you understand it.

Unsurprisingly, chronic stress can have a seriously negative impact on your health. For one thing, belly fat is associated with the development of cardiovascular disease and type 2 diabetes. The National Cholesterol Education Program states that a waist circumference of ≥35 inches for women and ≥40 inches for men is a risk factor for metabolic syndrome, a cluster of conditions that may lead to cardiovascular disease and type 2 diabetes. Also, when body tissues are exposed to high levels of cortisol for extended periods of time, some undesirable cellular and tissue alterations may occur. In addition, high blood pressure, elevated blood fats, and increased blood glucose have all been linked to elevated cortisol levels.

As you may already know, cortisol has become a prime subject of fascination, discussion, and confusion within the consumer and fitness industry, in large part due to misleading television commercials and advertisements. Some supplement manufacturers have created advertisements labeling cortisol as the villain hormone causing belly fat. And—wouldn't you know it?—these same companies sell products that supposedly counteract these bad effects. Unfortunately, this approach to resolving a person's accumulation of abdominal fat is futile. As discussed earlier, it is the *chronic stress* that is the issue here, not the cortisol. A person dealing with chronic stress doesn't need a cortisol-combatting product. Indeed, interventions to help this person deal with chronic stress are much more desirable. An effective and regular exercise and stress management program is the real key to better managing stress and in the long run, preventing stress-induced obesity.

WHAT CAN YOU DO ABOUT CHRONIC STRESS?

The first step to fighting chronic stress is to admit that you are having it. If you have been ignoring it, stop and face reality. Acknowledging that the stress is present is central to managing it. The second step involves problem solving. I always tell my students to be laser focused in their efforts to solve challenging problems. Try this. Laser focus on the best ways for you to deal with the chronic stressors in your life. Discussing your challenges with a colleague, friend, or mental health professional is often a productive way to figure out what is stressing you and how to overcome it. It's amazing how good you can be at problem solving when you laser focus on the RESOLUTION of the problem, and not just the problem.

Exercise is an outstanding stress management tool for treating stress-induced anxiety, so your HIIT workouts in this book should be a wonderful aid. Relaxation exercises may also help. Here's a simple breathing drill you can do any time to help lessen the effects of stress: sit very comfortably and focus on relaxing the muscles in your body, especially those that are tensing up. Keep your breathing very slow and controlled. As you inhale, say silently or out loud (depending on where you are), "I am." And as you exhale, say silently or out loud to yourself, "Calm." Continue this affirmation breathing exercise for 3–5 minutes. You can do this breathing drill at work, on a train or bus, in an airplane, at a restaurant, or pretty much anywhere you can give yourself a few minutes of time to focus. I do this affirmation breathing daily as I deal with my own stressors and can attest to how wonderfully it helps me manage stress. I am confident it will work just as well for you.

CHAPTER 15

50 Frequently Asked Health, Nutrition, and Weight Management Questions

At this point, hopefully you are raring to get up and HIIT the gym. (If so—I salute you!) Before we get to the workouts, though, I'd like to discuss some frequent hot-button topics. As a college professor, I get *a lot* of questions from my students related to weight management, exercise science, diet, exercise physiology, and health. I realized over time that many of the same questions were coming up again and again, so years ago I started keeping a record of my answers. I am certain that you have had at least some of these questions yourself, so I would like to share them with you. That said, if you just can't wait to HIIT it, feel free to skip ahead to the workouts. But make sure you come back to read these fifty most common questions about health, dieting, and exercise—and their evidence-based answers:

QUESTIONS ON HEALTH

1. **HOW DO I BOOST MY HDL CHOLESTEROL?** Your HDL cholesterol is the good or healthy cholesterol. It's the scavenger that travels through the blood and removes excess plaque that is starting to clog up your arteries. One major way to boost your HDL is to quit smoking, if you smoke. Quitting smoking has been shown to improve your HDL cholesterol and lower your LDL (bad) cholesterol. This is most impressive, as both of these changes reduce your

risk of cardiovascular disease. Definitely continue with your cardiorespiratory exercise. The HIIT workouts in this book are an excellent aerobic exercise program and have been shown to improve HDL cholesterol. Another great strategy to boost the effectiveness of HDL cholesterol is to replace saturated fats with healthier monounsaturated and polyunsaturated fats in your diet. And, if you drink, moderation is the key. (If you don't drink alcohol, though, don't start.) Lastly, I want to note that scientists believe that even if your HDL numbers do not go up, lifestyle modifications—such as the ones suggested in this book—can still improve your HDL cholesterol's functioning in the body. Your lifestyle behaviors can progressively improve components of the HDL cholesterol structure, making it a more potent plaque forager.

2. **WHAT ARE SOME WAYS TO BOOST MY ENERGY LEVEL?** Here are seven very effective tips for boosting your energy:

    a. Find a healthy balance with your diet and your physical activity. Very restrictive diets can make people feel fatigued during the day and sap their energy. In fact, some popular diets have been shown to be low in several micronutrients, including vitamin B7, vitamin D, vitamin E, chromium, iodine, and molybdenum. Being deficient in these nutrients can definitely cause your energy to be low.

    b. Make sure you are drinking enough water. The Institute of Medicine has determined that adequate water intake for men is roughly 13 cups (3 liters) a day, and the adequate intake for women is about 9 cups (2.2 liters) a day.

    c. Make sure you are getting enough healthy carbohydrates. Carbohydrates are the main energy source for your body, which breaks them down into glucose to keep your cells working well. Healthy whole grains, like those in whole grain bread and oatmeal, take longer to digest but give you sustained energy. Also, for more sustained energy, try adding a little protein to the carbohydrates, as this slows digestion further. Greek yogurt in particular is packed with protein, boasting 15 to 20 grams per six-ounce serving.

d. Keep an eye on iron. It's no secret that iron deficiency is a common cause of fatigue in women. Don't forget that tofu and kidney beans are good sources of this essential mineral, as is lean red meat.

e. Don't skip breakfast. It helps maintain blood sugar levels that have dropped during your previous evening of sleep.

f. Sleep on. It's important to get all the sleep your body needs. Losing only 1 or 2 hours can sap you in the middle of the day and even lead to weight gain. Strive for 6 to 8 hours of sleep nightly.

g. Exercise. Cardiorespiratory exercise and resistance training improve several metabolic processes in the body, leading to increased energy.

3. **IS IT OK TO DRINK BEER AFTER WORKING OUT?** Alcohol is a diuretic, which means it stimulates urine production. Following a workout, you want to *replenish* your body with lost fluids, not take more away from it. Consequently, drinking an alcoholic beverage before or after exercise is NOT recommended.

4. **CAN I DRINK TOO MUCH CAFFEINE?** Most people have internal regulators that tell them when to stop consuming caffeine. However, experts from the Mayo Clinic suggest up to 400 milligrams (mg) of caffeine a day—roughly the amount in four cups of brewed coffee—appears to be safe for most healthy adults. Be aware of the symptoms of "caffeinism": breathlessness, headache, lightheadedness, and irregular heartbeat. Too much caffeine may also trigger a panic attack. For college students, caffeine-containing energy drinks have overtaken coffee as the primary source of caffeine. If you decide to consume one of these drinks, please check the label to make sure your caffeine intake is within recommended levels.

5. **WHAT DOES IT MEAN WHEN A FOOD HAS THE AMERICAN HEART ASSOCIATION LOGO ON IT?** The red heart with white checkmark means the food has no more than 3 grams of fat, 20 milligrams of cholesterol, and 480 milligrams of sodium. The food must also have

at least 10 percent of the daily value for one or more of these nutrients: protein, vitamin A, vitamin C, calcium, iron, or dietary fiber.

6. **IS IT TRUE THAT TEA IS A HEALTHY BEVERAGE?** Yes, black and green teas appear to lessen cholesterol's damaging effect on your arteries and protect against cancers of the skin and gastrointestinal tract. If you drink tea, make sure you steep it for at least 3 minutes to ensure the beneficial antioxidants in the leaves enter your beverage.

7. **WHAT ARE TRANS-FATTY ACIDS AND WHY ARE THEY BAD FOR YOU?** Trans-fatty acids are unsaturated fats that have had hydrogen added to them, making them more saturated. This chemical process helps to extend the shelf life of many foods, such as crackers, cakes, cookies, chips, and unsaturated oils (such as corn and soybean). Regrettably, trans-fatty acids raise your total cholesterol and LDL (bad) cholesterol. They can also lower your HDL (healthy) cholesterol. In addition, trans fats are associated with increased risk of type 2 diabetes. When looking at food labels, the words "hydrogenated" and "partially hydrogenated" indicate there are trans fats in the food. Try to avoid these foods.

8. **IS THERE A DIFFERENCE BETWEEN BEING OVERFAT AND OVERWEIGHT?** Yes, overweight is a term that is only concerned with pounds. Overfat is concerned with the muscle/fat relationship. For instance, many professional football players are overweight by the familiar height/weight charts but have a low percentage of body fat, which means they are certainly not overfat.

9. **SHOULD I TAKE A MULTIVITAMIN?** Yes, this is an option to consider. Many people take a multivitamin because they are aware their diet is imperfect, which is a good reason to do so. If you take a multivitamin, make sure it has B12. Your body doesn't make B12, so you need to get it from animal-based foods (dairy products, eggs, fish, meat, and poultry) or from supplements. As you make the turn into your fifties, you absorb B12 less effectively. A B12 deficiency can lead to nerve damage. The average recommended amounts, measured in micrograms (mcg), is 2.4 mcg per day, 2.6 mcg per day if pregnant, and 2.8 mcg per day if breastfeeding. The other key vitamin to look for in a multivitamin is vitamin D.

Many Americans get too little vitamin D from sunlight or food. The recommended daily levels are 600 IU until age seventy and 800 IU if you are older than seventy. If you are already taking *some* vitamins, I recommend you talk with your health practitioner before starting a multivitamin, as too many vitamins can become toxic to your body. However, I describe taking a multivitamin as being similar to an insurance policy. It is a daily guarantee to ensure that your body gets the vitamins and minerals it needs. A multivitamin can make up for the shortfalls that happen when you don't get the nutrition you need through food.

10. **AM I AT INCREASED CANCER RISK IF I EAT RED MEAT?** Yes, according to research presented by the National Institutes of Health and National Cancer Institute. Eating a high consumption of red meat increases the likelihood of someone developing colorectal cancer. Minimize your intake of processed red meats such as sausage, hot dogs, bacon, and lunchmeats, as they have the strongest links to cancer development. Red meat consumption in early adult life for a woman is more associated with breast cancer risk than red meat consumption in midlife or later for a woman. Also, here's a note of safety for those of you who enjoy barbecuing your meats: cooking meat at high temperatures causes chemicals called heterocyclic amines (HCAs) to form. These HCAs are carcinogens that can cause changes in your DNA, which may lead to cancer. There are several ways to minimize HCAs when you grill. For starters, you can eliminate 90% of the HCAs if you microwave your meat or chicken first for about 1.5–2 minutes. Then, just pour off the juices. Turning over the meat and poultry every minute cuts the HCAs by 75–95% because the surface temperature stays lower. Remember, however, the drier and more well-done the meat, the more HCAs you get.

11. **ARE SWEET POTATO FRIES HEALTHIER THAT REGULAR FRENCH FRIES?** It seems like sweet potato fries are showing up on menus in many restaurants, which raises this common question. Sorry, but sweet potato fries are still fries. The name "sweet potato fries" sounds like a healthy alternative, but it really isn't—both are loaded with calories and sodium. A better side dish option is a green salad or non-starchy vegetables like asparagus or broccoli.

12. **IS IT POSSIBLE TO BE FAT BUT FIT?** The paradox of being fat but fit has stimulated quite a bit of interest in medicine and fitness, and it's an important phenomenon to discuss,

particularly as populations around the world are becoming more overweight. Dr. Jean-Pierre Després, the world acclaimed obesity and cardiovascular disease researcher from Université Laval in Quebec, Canada, has addressed the fat but fit issue in his research. He asserts that reducing waist circumference by increasing cardiorespiratory fitness with exercise and incorporating movement to combat sedentary behavior will result in positive health benefits, even in the absence of weight loss. Dr. Després points out that most people who are fat but fit are in the overweight/moderately obese range; they are not vastly obese. Fat but fit individuals tend to have less belly fat, the unhealthy danger zone for fat accumulation on your body. (As a reminder, HIIT exercise programs have been shown to selectively target unhealthy belly fat.) Finally, changing from a sedentary behavior to a physically active lifestyle is the major key when discussing this fat but fit question. In summary: yes, you can be fat but fit!

13. **ARE NUTS REALLY THAT HEALTHY?** Absolutely. A recent study published in the *New England Journal of Medicine* followed 119,000 women and men for twenty-four years, and found that adults who regularly consume nuts were less likely to die of heart disease, cancer, and lung disease. Nuts are rich in unsaturated fats, protein, vitamin E, and fiber, and low in carbohydrates. Other studies have shown that nuts can improve blood pressure and cholesterol and reduce the risk of type 2 diabetes. This new study suggests that for optimal results you should eat a handful of nuts a day, which is about 3 tablespoons (or one ounce). Nuts pack a few calories (160–204 calories per ounce), but the research does not indicate you are going to get fat from eating them. Still, it is good to be aware of this if you are on a weight management plan, as nuts do add to your caloric intake. Also, the thousands of men and women in this study ate all types of nuts, as well as peanuts, which is actually a legume. However, the researchers suggest that walnuts, almonds, and hazelnuts are particularly recommended for cardiovascular health. Here are some "nutty" ideas to consider for your daily life: instead of snacking on sweets or chips, replace them with a handful of your favorite nuts. Also, top green salads with nuts instead of cheese or meats. Another great option is to sprinkle some nuts on your favorite yogurt. Make sure you store nuts properly, as they can go bad. Keep them in an airtight container in your refrigerator or a sealed plastic bag in your freezer.

14. **WHAT IS THE BODY MASS INDEX (BMI) MEASUREMENT I'VE READ ABOUT IN WEIGHT MANAGEMENT ARTICLES?** BMI is calculated as your weight in kilograms divided by the square of your height (in meters). Another simple BMI calculation is body weight in pounds multiplied by 703 and then divided by height in inches. Fortunately, there are many easy-to-use BMI calculators on the web. The World Health Organization has established guidelines for normal (18.5–24.9 kg/m^2), overweight (25–29.9 kg/m^2) and obese (>30 kg/m^2) BMI in adults. One of the drawbacks of BMI, though, is that a muscular person will score higher, producing an inaccurate assessment that they are overweight or obese. Also, studies indicate that older people tend to lose muscle mass, possibly leading to an underestimate of the BMI. As we have discussed in this book, the ever-increasing worldwide obesity epidemic poses increased risk for coronary heart disease, hypertension, abnormal cholesterol, type 2 diabetes, sleep apnea, and certain cancers. This helps explain the popularity of BMI, which is a simple measurement tool for identifying people at risk. More recently, however, waist circumference has been used to identify health risks for obesity in place of BMI. A waist circumference ≥35 inches in women and ≥40 inches in men is associated with higher cardiovascular disease risk. One practical question you probably have is, how is waist circumference measured? Hold the tape snugly right around your belly button. It is that easy. Go ahead—measure yourself when you're ready. I encourage my students to track their waist circumference every 2 months after they start their HIIT workouts to see what changes are occurring here.

15. **WHAT CAN I DO TO PREVENT MYSELF FROM GETTING CARDIOVASCULAR DISEASE?** This is the perfect question to finish this health section. If I could get everyone to follow the following guidelines, we would be able to celebrate a magnificent reduction in cardiovascular disease throughout the world. Here are the top ten evidence-based strategies to prevent cardiovascular disease.

a. Do not smoke. If you don't smoke, don't start. Those who smoke have a seven-fold increase in risk.

b. Stay active, and keep it brisk. The evidence is crystal clear that physically active people have a lower risk of heart disease. But it's important to challenge yourself, too! Be sure that whatever activity you do gets progressively more challenging. The better your cardiovascular health, the lower your disease risk. Remember, for every 30 minutes of sitting, get your 3 minutes (or more) of movement.

c. Check your weight regularly. Being overweight increases the risk of being obese. And, obesity increases the risk for cardiovascular disease. Use the weight management strategies in this book to put yourself on the road to optimal health, fitness, and quality of life.

d. Keep your blood pressure under control. High blood pressure intensifies the risk of a heart attack more in women than it does in men, but it is vitally important for men to have healthy blood pressure, too. Ideally, you want a systolic blood pressure under 120mmHg and diastolic under 80mmHg. Following a heart-healthy diet and exercise plan is the best way to manage blood pressure.

d. Go heart-healthy. The American Heart Association encourages you to eat fatty fish 2 to 3 times a week to get those very healthy omega-3 fats. If you eat meat, just select smaller portion sizes. Eat plenty of fruits, nuts, beans, vegetables, and whole grains. Definitely choose unsaturated fats, which come from foods like avocados, seeds, nuts, and vegetable oils. Avoid and/or minimize sugary foods and refined carbohydrates. Reduce your intake of processed foods that have those undesirable hydrogenated oils and trans fats.

e. Keep sodium consumption down. Watch out for the big three here: processed food, restaurant meals, and fast food. See if you can cut back on one, two, or all three.

f. If you drink, drink moderately. Moderate drinking is not more than two drinks a day for men and one drink a day for women. That is doable.

g. Manage your stress. Chronic stress can be enormously disruptive, psychologically and physiologically. If you need help, go get it!

h. Monitor your cholesterol. Have your health practitioner check your LDL (bad) cholesterol and HDL (good) cholesterol regularly. This information gives you some useful knowledge when it comes to knowing how well your body's cardioprotection is shielding you from cardiovascular events.

i. Have your blood sugar checked. Men and women with moderately elevated blood sugar—what we call "prediabetes"—are at a higher risk of cardiovascular disease. At yearly health checkups, where you get to monitor your cholesterol, be sure to also have your blood sugar measured and checked.

One final thought on heart disease. It is always helpful to be aware of any family history of heart disease, since it is a disease that runs in families. Discovering that it's part of your family history may make you more aggressive in following the preventative strategies I described above. You are in control!

QUESTIONS ON NUTRITION

16. **IS IT OK IF I DRINK SMOOTHIES?** Several franchises now sell many types of smoothies, or "functional beverages," as we academic types like to call them. Most of these smoothies are made from fruit, juice, milk, yogurt, sorbet, and special "boosts" of herbs, vitamins, fiber, protein, and other substances. Some of the claims made by these businesses are pretty outlandish, suggesting the drinks can control stress, improve mood, and increase energy. However, smoothies made from melons, carrots, berries, and other produce truly do have healthy minerals, vitamins, fiber, and phytochemicals. Phytochemicals are quite beneficial for human health and in preventing diseases. Some of the phytochemicals from plant foods can neutralize those unsafe free radicals that we talked about earlier in the book. The downside of some of these smoothies is that they pack a lot of calories; some have 500 to 700 calories per smoothie, which may very well contribute to weight gain. So, although healthful for the most part, they may not be the best for a weight management program.

17. **WHY ARE FOODS WITH HYDROGENATED OILS BAD FOR ME?** The problem with hydrogenated oils is they contain trans fats, which raise the bad LDL cholesterol and lower the good HDL cholesterol. In the hydrogenation process, hydrogen atoms are added to a vegetable oil's available bonds. Unfortunately, as the level of hydrogenation increases, the level of saturated fat also increases. I encourage you to read food labels. If the ingredient list contains the words "hydrogenated" or "partially hydrogenated," the food contains trans fats, and you should steer clear. Foods that often contain trans fats include fried fast foods, cakes, cookies (particularly with frosting), pies, doughnuts, baked goods, frozen biscuits, breakfast sandwiches, crackers, microwave popcorn, frozen pizza, and some margarines. As you may know, the process of hydrogenation extends the shelf life of a product, thus saving money for the company that produces it. Good for them, perhaps, but not good for you.

18. **DO VITAMINS GIVE ME EXTRA ENERGY?** This is a very popular question that I get all of the time. Unlike carbohydrates, fats, and proteins, vitamins do not provide usable energy. I tell my students that vitamins are the worker bees in metabolism, because they assist enzymes in releasing energy from carbohydrates, fats, and proteins. However, vitamins are almost entirely calorie free.

19. **WHAT ARE THE BEST FOODS TO EAT AFTER ONE OF MY HIIT WORKOUTS?** First and foremost, focus on replenishing lost water after your workout. So start by hydrating. Next, select a food rich in complex carbohydrates (starches, not sugars) and some protein. For instance, you could have a peanut butter and banana sandwich, or hummus and tomato on pita bread, or half a turkey wrap with veggies.

20. **WHAT IS DIETARY FIBER?** Dietary fiber is basically a type of complex carbohydrate made up of plant material that cannot be digested by the human body. Refining and processing foods removes almost all of its natural fiber. The main sources of dietary fiber are whole grain cereals and breads, fruits, and vegetables. Optimal amounts of fiber in the diet increase gastric movement and therefore may reduce the incidence of diverticulosis (bulging sacs or small blisters that appear in the lining of your large intestine), colon and rectal cancer, and obesity.

21. **ARE NATURAL VITAMINS BETTER FOR ME THAN MANUFACTURED VITAMINS?** No. For the most part your body can't distinguish the difference between vitamins manufactured in a laboratory and natural vitamins extracted from food. So if you get a cold, go ahead and eat oranges and other vitamin C-rich fruits *and* get plenty of supplemental vitamin C.

22. **WHAT IS THE DIFFERENCE BETWEEN BROWN RICE AND WHITE RICE?** Brown rice has slightly more vitamin E, magnesium, and some other minerals. The nutty flavor and chewy texture of brown rice is due to retention of the grain's bran. Brown rice also has more grams of fiber than white rice.

23. **WHAT'S THE FINAL SCOOP: BUTTER OR MARGARINE?** Good question. According to the Mayo Clinic, margarine usually tops butter. Butter is made from animal fat, so it contains more saturated fat. However, stick margarines contain trans fats to keep them solid. As I've mentioned, trans fats can increase your risk of heart disease. The best advice is to look for a soft tub margarine that doesn't have trans fats and has the least amount of saturated fat. Another option would be to spread your bread with olive oil. Olive oil is a monounsaturated fatty acid, which is considered a healthy fat. Try it and see if you like it. I use it all the time!

24. **WHAT IS THE MOST COMMON NUTRITIONAL DEFICIENCY IN THE UNITED STATES?** Iron deficiency. Despite iron's abundance on earth, iron deficiency is surprisingly common in humans and is the prevailing cause of anemia throughout the world. It affects some eight million women of childbearing age and upward of seven hundred thousand toddlers. Iron deficiency anemia happens when your body doesn't have enough iron to make hemoglobin. Hemoglobin is the part of red blood cells that gives blood its red color and helps the red blood cells carry oxygen throughout your body. Examples of iron-rich foods include leafy green vegetables, iron-fortified foods, meat, and eggs.

25. **ARE PHYTONUTRIENTS THE SAME AS PHYTOCHEMICALS?** Yes, phytonutrients are phytochemicals. These unique nutrients are concentrated in the skins of many vegetables and fruits, and are responsible for their color, scent, and flavor. Phytochemicals are not vitamins

or minerals, however, they are plant nutrients that offer great health benefits. They have been shown to protect against heart disease, cancer, diabetes, osteoporosis, and other medical conditions. The only way to get phytochemicals is to eat or drink them in fruits, vegetables, juices, nuts, and whole grain products. Foods that are rich in phytochemicals include grapes, red cabbages, sweet potatoes, broccoli, kale, tomatoes, red onions, green tea, parsley, spinach, blueberries, raspberries, blackberries, and melons. The best-known phytochemicals are flavonoids, carotenoids, polyphenols, indoles, lignans, and isoflavones. Do you recognize any of these names?

26. **CAN VEGETARIANS GET ENOUGH PROTEIN?** Yes, vegetarians who eat a wide variety of foods each day will absorb a full complement of essential amino acids. Essential amino acids are the protein building blocks your body is unable to synthesize on its own, so we get these from our foods we eat. Nuts, seeds, legumes, and many grains are good sources of amino acids.

27. **WHY ARE WHOLE GRAINS BETTER THAN REFINED GRAINS?** Refined grains include white bread, white rice, regular white pasta, and other foods that have been made with white flour. Many cookies, cakes, breakfast cereals, crackers, and snack foods are also made of refined grains. Whole grains consist of the entire grain. They still contain the bran and germ, which are rich in dietary fiber and micronutrients. Whole grains are associated with a lower risk of cardiovascular disease, cancer, and all causes of mortality. Go with whole grains!

28. **WHAT SUGGESTIONS DO YOU HAVE FOR CHOOSING VEGGIE BURGERS?** Buyers beware. Even though veggie burgers are made of veggies, the amount of processing these ingredients go through may zap most of the essential nutrients from them. Start by checking the sodium level. Some veggie burgers have 500 (or more) milligrams of sodium, which is a third of your day's recommended total. Try to choose a veggie burger that has 350 milligrams or less. Next, check the protein in the veggie burger. In a 3-ounce beef burger you will get about 20 grams of protein. The protein in veggie burgers ranges from 5 to 20 grams, so shoot for one that has at least 10 grams of protein. The good news is most veggie burgers are

made with soybean oil, corn oil, or canola oil, all of which have more polyunsaturated fat, the good fat. Stay away from veggie burgers with Quorn. The main ingredient in Quorn is mycoprotein, which is a processed mold that can lead to very unhealthy reactions for some people. Alas, taste is the last decision. That is completely up to you.

29. AS I START WORKING OUT HARDER, WOULD IT BE BENEFICIAL TO HAVE A PRE-EXERCISE SNACK? A pre-exercise snack may be helpful if you feel like you don't have energy to complete your HIIT workouts. However, pre-exercise snacks have calories, and thus may thwart some of your weight management goals. Nevertheless, here's the scoop on pre-exercise snacks: muscle glycogen (the stored form of glucose, or sugar) is the principal fuel used by the body during exercise, followed by fat. This is primarily because we break down carbohydrates about thirty to forty times faster than we break down fat for energy, and during exercise we need energy rapidly to keep up with the HIIT workout. Low muscle glycogen stores may result in muscle fatigue and the body's inability to complete your HIIT workouts, particularly as you do the more challenging workouts. So, the demand for carbohydrates is relatively high for all types of challenging exercise. A carbohydrate and protein snack or drink prior to aerobic exercise has been shown to increase performance during challenging workouts. If you feel you need more energy for your workouts, try this approach: In choosing a supplement drink or snack, choose one with 3 to 4 units of carbohydrate to 1 unit of protein. We call this a 3/1 carbohydrate-to-protein ratio or a 4/1 carbohydrate-to-protein ratio; many health food stores have sports drinks and snacks you can try with these ratios. I recommended you have your drink or snack within 30 minutes of exercise. See if this helps give you the energy to sustain your workouts.

30. I AM THINKING OF SNACKING ON NUTRITION BARS BETWEEN SOME OF MY REGULAR MEALS. WHAT DO I NEED TO KNOW TO CHOOSE THE RIGHT ONE? Nutrition bars are also called "energy bars." They offer wonderful convenience and variety and can be a snack, protein booster, nutritional supplement, or even a meal replacement. They also travel well. Before choosing a nutrition bar, though, consider that they contain an average of 150 to 300 calories. For a person on a weight-loss program that is *a lot*! If you are on a weight management program, seek a lower-calorie bar. Also, even though they have the word "nutrition" on the label, many of these bars are packed with sweeteners, such as high fructose corn syrup, honey, molasses, and cane sugar. Sugar is sugar, which means there really isn't any nutritional value to any of these sugars, just extra calories. Try to avoid nutrition bars with processed sugars such as fructose, sucrose, and dextrose. Cranberries, dates, figs, apricots, raisins, and other dried fruits are healthier sweeteners in nutrition bars. When it comes to protein, many nutrition bars have 10 to 15 grams of protein, often from whey protein, which is a dairy source. Some bars get their protein from seeds, legumes, and nuts. You probably don't need that much protein, but protein does promote satiety, so you will feel full for a longer period of time. Steer away from soy protein isolate, which may act as a hormone disruptor in the body. In regard to fat, check to see if the bar has the favorable unsaturated fats, including canola oil, sunflower oil, nuts, and seeds. Steer away from nutrition bars that have saturated fats such as palm oil, coconut oil, and cocoa butter. In addition, most nutrition bars have 3 to 5 grams of fiber, which is healthful. Many nutrition bars have about 100 to 150 milligrams of sodium, which is fine for this kind of a snack. Moreover, many nutrition bars have an array of added nutrients, such as vitamin E, vitamin C, beta-carotene, folic acid, copper, and magnesium. That said, if you are eating a healthy diet you may not need any more of these nutrients. Now that you know how to recognize a healthy nutrition bar, the last step is making sure you find a brand and flavor that tastes good to you. It's best to buy different bars separately, as opposed to in a box, so you can try them out first. Some health food stores also let you buy a sampler box of different bars to better make your final choices. Healthy snacking!

31. **I AM THINKING OF SWITCHING TO NONDAIRY MILK. WHAT SHOULD I LOOK FOR WHEN I BUY IT?** Many Americans have made the switch from cow's milk to "milks" made from cashews, almonds, flax, hemp oats, rice, soy, and other plants. As a result, the nondairy milk market is booming. Here are some tips in making your selection for nondairy milk. In regard to protein, cow's milk has 8 grams of protein per cup of milk. Most of your plant options are much lower, coming in closer to 1 gram per cup. However, soy milk delivers protein levels similar to cow's milk. Make sure you check the label if protein is one of the macronutrients you are seeking. Cow's milk has plenty of calcium, potassium, vitamin D, and vitamin B12. Check for these nutrients in the nondairy options. Please don't be fooled

by the big calcium claims in some of these nondairy milks. The calcium Recommended Dietary Allowance (RDA) for adults is 1,000 milligrams per day, and 1,200 milligrams for women over fifty and men over seventy. Too much calcium, however, puts you at risk for hip fractures and kidney stones. More calcium is not better! Also watch out for the sugar in nondairy options. Cow's milk has 12 grams of natural sugar (called "lactose"), which is about 3 teaspoons. Try the unsweetened nondairy milk options or some of the "original" nondairy milk options such as original soy or almond milk. An ingredient in some nondairy milk to avoid is carrageenan, which has been shown to cause long-lasting digestive problems. Guar gum and xanthan gum are two other substances often found in nondairy milks that you should avoid; they have been linked to digestive problems and weight gain. Lastly, most nondairy milks are low in saturated (bad) fat.

32. **PLEASE CLARIFY: IT IS NOW OK TO EAT EGGS?** That is correct. The Dietary Guidelines Advisory Committee has concluded that cholesterol in foods such as eggs is NOT the main cause of unhealthy blood cholesterol levels. Now, this isn't a green light to eat as many eggs as you want. But, having a couple of eggs every other day is fine. However, please use moderation if you have bacon, sausage, and/or ham with your eggs, as those processed meats are highly linked to cancer and heart disease.

QUESTIONS ON WEIGHT MANAGEMENT

33. **WHAT'S A GOOD SUBSTITUTE FOR THOSE HIGH-FAT POTATO CHIP SNACKS?** Try pretzels. They're almost fat free. If you are intent on buying chips, look for the chips that are baked, not fried, and avoid chips made in hydrogenated oil. Remember to check the total fat content and serving size, too.

34. **ARE THERE ANY FOODS THAT WILL MAKE ME MORE SATISFIED AND LESS LIKELY TO BINGE?** Yes. Some of the most filling foods include boiled potatoes, steamed fish, oatmeal, oranges, apples, whole wheat pasta, grilled lean beef, baked beans, grapes, and whole grain bread.

35. **WHAT IS GRAZING?** Grazing is an eating plan some people have adopted where they eat frequent small meals (up to six) spaced throughout the day. Some people find that this helps control appetite, and they actually consume fewer calories than if they had eaten three square meals. The one downside of this eating plan is the time it takes to plan, prepare, and then eat the smaller meals.

36. **IS IT TRUE THAT WHEN YOU EAT OUT, YOU USUALLY EAT MORE CALORIES THAN AT HOME?** Yes. Large portion sizes and high-calorie entrees carry most of this responsibility. Be aware that when you go out you are almost always less likely to eat nutritious food. Also remember that appetizers (which means "small dishes") have calories, too. Alas, most Americans neglect fruits and vegetables when eating out.

37. **ARE LIQUID MEAL REPLACEMENTS OK TO TAKE ON A REGULAR BASIS?** Many of these liquid meals provide sufficient calories as well as a number of minerals and vitamins, but they do not provide the health-promoting fiber and phytochemicals that are in fruits and vegetables. So, I don't mean to discourage their consumption, but make sure you balance them with real meals, fruits, and vegetables.

38. **I LIKE ORANGE JUICE WITH PULP. DOES IT HAVE MORE FIBER THAN JUICE WITHOUT PULP?** There is no significant difference in the fiber content between juice with pulp and juice without it. The pulp is composed of specialized cells that help store the juice.

39. **CAN I REDUCE THE NUMBER OF FAT CELLS IN MY BODY?** No, you can reduce the *size* of the fat cells, but not their number. Woefully, you can certainly increase the number of fat cells. Continual weight gain will lead to the expansion of existing fat cells and the creation of more cells. Once created, these new fat cells will not go away!

40. **WHAT IS THE INTUITIVE EATING DIET?** Intuitive eating is a dietary strategy that encourages you to listen and respond to your body's hunger signals for food choices. The view of this non-diet approach is to encourage normal, healthy, and conscious eating. Intuitive eating has an empowering philosophy to be more mindful at meal times. This enables people

to trust themselves in what they eat and how much they eat. Study results indicate that intuitive eating promotes heightened awareness and responses to body signals that result in healthy, long-term behavior change. Try this—it works for many people.

41. **WHY DOES THE MIRROR SHOW THE CHANGE OF MY SHAPE BEFORE THE SCALE?** Great observation. Muscle is denser than fat. A pound of fat bulges out 18% more than a pound of muscle. Because you are adding muscle to your body as you shape up, you will often notice a loss of inches before a loss of weight.

42. **WHAT ROLE DOES GENETICS PLAY WHEN IT COMES TO WEIGHT MANAGEMENT?** It is now well established that being overweight and obesity are conditions that tend to concentrate within a family. The risk for obesity is two to eight times higher for a person with a family history of obesity, as opposed to a person with no family history of obesity. However, genes do not always predict the future. A person's susceptibility for obesity derives from a lifestyle of abundant food intake in combination with little exercise. Obesity is definitely preventable.

43. **WILL EATING SPICY FOODS HELP ME BURN MORE CALORIES?** Spicy foods such as red or green chili peppers contain capsaicin, a chemical compound that can mildly boost your metabolism. Some studies suggest the effect only lasts about half an hour, however. Therefore, in the long run, eating lots of spicy food is not an effective weight management strategy.

44. **WHAT CAN I DO TO AVOID EATING TOO MUCH JUNK FOOD?** One of the first steps to avoiding junk food is to not get too hungry between meals. There are so many irresistible food cues from fast food enticing you to eat it when you are hungry. Make a list of healthy snacks that you can enjoy if you get hungry between meals, and choose these first. For some people, daily stressors sometimes prompt the consumption of junk food. Be aware of this and have some healthy stress-relief solutions at the ready. Also, laser focus on always eating the healthiest foods for your body, and make sure you have healthy snacks readily available when you are experiencing cravings.

45. I REALIZE CUTTING SUGAR-SWEETENED BEVERAGES IS IMPORTANT FOR WEIGHT CONTROL. WHY HAVE THESE DRINKS BECOME SUCH A PROBLEM? The consumption of soft drinks, sodas, and sugar-sweetened beverages has been increasing in almost every country in the world. This is an alarming trend, given the strong evidence linking drinking sugary drinks and weight gain, particularly when it comes to children. Accordingly, limiting the consumption of sugar-sweetened beverages has a particularly central role in weight management. A typical 20-ounce soda has 15 to 18 teaspoons of sugar and over 240 calories. A 64-ounce fountain soda drink could have up to 700 calories. Why are people drinking these? Research studies suggest people who drink sugar-sweetened drinks do not feel as full as they would have if they had eaten the same number of calories from solid food. Therefore, they do not compensate by eating less food. Fundamentally, these sugar-sweetened sodas deliver a pack of calories with sugar dissolved in water, which our bodies do not compensate for by eating less of other foods. And, regrettably, these sugar-sweetened drinks have little to no nutritional value. The best advice is to start substituting water for sugary sodas. Start slowly, remembering your slogan (the same one that applies to all of the changes proposed in this book): "Inch by inch, it's a cinch."

46. IS THERE ANY RESEARCH SUGGESTING ALTERNATE-DAY FASTING IS A VIABLE OPTION TO TRY FOR WEIGHT LOSS? Alternate-day fasting is a new approach for weight loss. It's meant to address the reality that many people just do not like to reduce their calories on a daily basis. With the alternate-day fasting approach, participants restrict calories every other day. This strategy involves a fast day when you consume 25% of your usual intake, approximately 500 calories. The fast day alternates with a feast day when you are permitted to consume food at your pleasure—whatever you feel. There are several published books on this approach and a few 2–3 month studies that show impressive 3% to 7% drops in body weight among people who used this strategy. These short-term studies also show improvements in blood pressure, blood fats and the body's ability to use glucose for fuel. A 2017 study published in the *JAMA Internal Medicine,* compared alternate-day fasting to a traditional caloric restriction diet for a one-year period, with one hundred men and women, eighteen to sixty-five years of age. At 6 months both groups had lost approximately 7% body weight and at 12 months both groups pretty much maintained their loss in body weight. Also, by 12 months there were no differences between the two groups when it came to changes in blood pressure, blood fats and glucose metabolism. The researchers concluded that alternate-day fasting was equivalent to daily caloric restriction for weight loss, weight maintenance, and cardioprotection. So, alternate-day fasting appears to be an effective weight management approach that may be of interest to you.

47. **IS THERE EVIDENCE TO SUPPORT THE CLAIM THAT A GLUTEN-FREE DIET IS GOOD FOR WEIGHT LOSS?** Gluten-free diets are one of the newer weight loss crazes endorsed by celebrities and supported by a surge of internet articles and books. To understand more about these diets, let's start by exploring celiac disease. According to the Celiac Disease Foundation, celiac disease is an autoimmune disorder in which the ingestion of gluten leads to damage in the small intestine. This hereditary disease is estimated to impact one in one hundred people worldwide. When a person with celiac disease eats gluten, a protein found in wheat, rye and barley, his or her body's immune system attacks the lining of the small intestine. This causes pain, bloating, cramps, diarrhea and eventual vitamin deficiencies. Gluten acts like glue that holds food together, and thus can be found in many types of foods. People on a gluten-free diet must avoid foods with any trace of wheat, rye, or barley. Wheat is found in breads, soups, baked goods, pasta, cereals, salad dressing, and sauces. Barley is found in food coloring, soups, beer, malt and brewer's yeast. Rye is found in rye bread, pumpernickel bread and some cereals. Fortunately for people with celiac disease, there is an ever-increasing market of gluten-free products that can help them enjoy a satisfying lifestyle. But, the question many people have is, will a gluten-free lifestyle melt down the pounds? A rigorous search for randomized control studies (the most effective investigations) focusing on gluten-free eating and weight loss indicates a lack of research on this topic at present. Nevertheless, whenever anyone goes on a restrictive diet, she/he typically eats less, which may explain why some people have lost weight on a gluten-free diet. But be forewarned, many gluten-free products on the market have higher proportions of fats and proteins. So, if you go gluten-free, keep an eye on your calorie intake.

48. I KNOW I NEED TO CUT DOWN ON SALT, BUT HOW DO I DO THIS? Most Americans eat more than the recommended 2,300 milligrams of daily sodium. Sodium's fundamental role is to help muscles and nerves work efficiently. If you are able to eat less salt by choosing low-sodium foods, this will likely lower your blood pressure if it is elevated, or better manage your current blood pressure. It is important to note that high blood pressure is associated with heart disease, stroke, congestive heart failure, and kidney disease. You get a whopping 80% of your dietary salt from eating at restaurants or preprepared, processed meals. So, be aware of this. Also, there are many spice substitutes you can try instead of salt. For meats, poultry, soups and sauces, try spicing things up with cayenne pepper, allspice, chili powder, cilantro, or paprika. For salads and vegetables, try parsley, sage, thyme and cinnamon. Enjoy!

49. I SEE A NUMBER OF ADVERTISEMENTS FOR "FAT BURNER" PRODUCTS. DO ANY OF THEM WORK? Dietary supplement manufacturers often use the term "fat burner" to describe supplements or products that supposedly speed up your body's metabolism of fat and calories. The manufacturers of these products claim the unique combination of substances in their special pill or powder provides a weight loss effect on your body. Some of the most popular fat burners include the following ingredients: carnitine, caffeine, conjugated linoleic acid, green tea, forskolin, chromium, kelp, and fucoxanthin. These products have little rigorous scientific proof for their claims. The scientist in me would like to discuss all of these ingredients with you, but, the practitioner in me will get straight to the bottom line: please save your money on these advertised fat burner products for now. Although a few products show some promise, more research is needed before you can get enthusiastic about using them. A much better—and rigorously tested—solution is to start moving more every day, do your HIIT workouts, and find a healthy dietary strategy that works for you!

50. WILL I BURN MORE CALORIES FROM FAT IF I EXERCISE FIRST THING IN THE MORNING ON AN EMPTY STOMACH? No. This question has been controversial in the fitness industry for decades. Some fitness gurus have been proclaiming that to lose more fat people should exercise in the morning in a fasted state. The research, however, clearly refutes this claim. Indeed, if you want to burn more calories you should eat a light breakfast or snack prior to your morning workout. In fact, the research shows that when you have a light breakfast prior to your workout, you actually burn more fat and more total calories over the 24 hours *after* the workout. WOW! Try this approach: have a light breakfast of some fruits, whole grain cereal, an energy bar, or a sports drink at least 20 to 30 minutes and up to 1 hour before your morning workout. Doing this before your morning workout will help you get some fuel in your tank for burning more calories and burning fat.

SECTION 3

Let's HIIT the Workouts!

Pre-Exercise Fundamentals

I WANT YOU TO REALLY ENJOY EXERCISE AND COMMIT TO MAKING IT A PART OF YOUR lifestyle. Before you jump in, however, I want to briefly go over some guidelines that will help ensure that your exercise program is safe and fruitful.

GET PHYSICIAN CLEARANCE BEFORE STARTING YOUR WORKOUTS

Any type of exercise is challenging to your body. Since I cannot individually screen you to determine your current fitness level, as a first and very important step, please check with your physician or health practitioner before starting these exercise workouts. It's important for you to get a clearance from your doctor before you begin any new—or different—type of exercise training program. Doing so will ensure that you are ready to embark on your new life of fitness and health. And if you're not ready yet, your doctor can help you figure out how to get ready.

WEAR PROPER EXERCISE GEAR FOR YOUR HIIT WORKOUTS

Every one of the HIIT workouts in this book can be done on almost any piece of aerobic exercise equipment. This versatility is one of the great advantages of HIIT training—it offers something for every enthusiast. This means each workout can be done walking, jogging, running, biking, elliptical striding, swimming, rowing, stair stepping, and/or on any type of cardio machine. Whatever exercise mode you select, take care in choosing your workout gear, because it will definitely influence the success of your workout. Your exercise clothing should be all about fit and comfort. If you decide to buy some new outfits, go ahead and choose clothing with some of your favorite colors. Yes—I want you to enjoy these workouts in fitness gear that functions well, looks great, and empowers you to exercise. If you plan on biking and/or swimming, make sure you get the specific types of clothing for these activities. For most of your other workouts, choose exercise gear that fits well and allows you to stay cool. Some light, breathable exercise-friendly fabrics with good stretch are nylon, polyester, spandex, and bamboo pulp. Cotton and cotton blend clothing is fine if you don't sweat that much; however, when you do sweat a lot, cotton clothing sticks to the body and becomes heavy. I often encourage fitness enthusiasts to go to a sporting goods store if there's one in their area, since this will allow you to see some of the different workout clothing options and try them on for fit. This also gives you a chance to speak with a qualified sales representative who may have good opinions on what works (and what doesn't). Make sure you wear supportive undergarments, such as a support bra, while doing your workouts. Undergarments provide support, lessen discomfort, and allow movement flexibility. Depending on the season and where you live, you may need to add a little layering if you exercise outside during the winter, or even during early morning or late evenings workouts during fall and spring.

YOUR FOOTWEAR BOOSTS THE WORKOUTS

When it comes to footwear, particularly new exercise shoes, I encourage fitness enthusiasts to go to a specialty sports shoe store where you can get guidance from knowledgeable staff. They can measure your feet and inspect your walking pattern and make some well-educated suggestions on what exercise footwear selections will work best for you. I always encourage enthusiasts to buy shoes later in the day, since your feet expand a little throughout the day. Your foot size changes as you age, so it is worth it to have both feet measured, even if you think you know your size. Did you know your feet swell after you walk, jog, or run? Yes, that's true. So, to find the best-fitting workout shoe, it would be good to do one of those activities for at least 10 minutes prior to buying. Definitely bring the type of sock you'll be wearing during exercise to your footwear fitting. If you wear orthotics, bring them along as well. Always walk and/or jog around the store a little while wearing the new shoes. The shoes should feel comfortable right away. I encourage students to get a workout shoe with a thumb's width between your big toe and the front end of the shoe. The shoe heel should fit snugly and provide good cushion. With your shoes on, take the "toe wiggle test." Here's how you do it: in a standing position, you should be able to wiggle all of your toes, on both feet. If you can do this, chances are you have the right fit. Some shoe experts suggest that a good fitness shoe can last up to 400 miles of walking and/or running. That may be true, but I always encourage exercise enthusiasts to invest in a new pair of shoes when the sole is worn out or the shoes start losing their support and comfort.

YOU NEED A WORKOUT TIMER

Lastly, let's talk timing. All of the HIIT workouts are timed for different lengths in seconds, minutes, or a combination of both. Lucky for you, there are many app timers on the market that provide precise timing and cool sound effect cues for your workout intervals. To select your personal app, just do a search for "interval training," "circuit training," or "HIIT training" apps on your smart phone. You will see many apps, all with multiple functions and options. Then select the timer you prefer.

Why Your Workout Warm-Up and Cooldown Are So Important

ALL OF THE GREAT HIIT WORKOUTS IN THIS BOOK HAVE BEEN ADAPTED FROM ACTUAL research studies. So it's worth noting that in each study, the participants included warm-up exercises that increased in intensity before their HIIT workout trials, and also had cooldown exercises after them. Scientists realize the body needs a progressive start before it can perform at its best, and it also needs to gradually taper down to pre-exercise levels of intensity after a workout is over. To find out more about why warm-ups and cooldowns are critical, and to see examples of pre-workout and post-workout exercises, please read on.

THE WARM-UP: PREPARE THE BODY AND TURN ON FAT BURNING

At the start of each HIIT workout I want you to do a 5–7 minute warm-up to adequately prepare your entire body for the exercises you are about to do. The warm-up should gradually progress in intensity, from a very light to a mild intensity. Students regularly ask me what happens to the body during the warm-up, and why is it so important? With that in mind, I'd like to highlight for you some of the really neat bodily responses that occur during the warm-up. As its name implies, the warm-up begins by eliciting a mild warming change in muscle temperature. This change helps your muscles contract more efficiently during the workout. Next, there's an internal shift of blood flow in your body to the muscles used in the warm-up. Your body is diverting blood from areas like the digestive system to the exercising muscles, and this increased blood flow is delivering more oxygen to the moving muscles. Not surprisingly, the warm-up boosts your heart rate and blood pressure, which helps to transport oxygen to those active muscles more effectively. Increasing oxygen to the exercising muscles is a marvelous mechanism for fat burning, since for muscles to burn fat, oxygen has to be available. In summary, the warm-up really helps the body gear up for burning fat during your workout.

The slight change in muscle temperature often produces some early sweating. This is helpful, as it gets your body's heat regulating mechanisms working properly. As you can tell, the warm-up is an important part of a great workout, with many bodily responses working together like a team to prepare you for the activity to come.

You may now be wondering, what's the best type of warm-up for my HIIT workouts? Without a doubt, the best warm-up is 5–7 minutes of the same exercise you will be doing, but at a light intensity. For instance, if you are doing a walking HIIT workout, then easy walking is the best warm-up. If you are doing a rowing HIIT workout, then light rowing is the best warm-up.

THE WORKOUT COOLDOWN: CALMING YOUR BODY AND MIND

The cooldown is the progressive recovery after your HIIT workout. It brings all the bodily processes that have been elevated by the workout (heart rate, blood pressure, breathing rate, and body temperature) slowly back down to pre-exercise levels. A good cooldown ensures that your blood returns safely and effectively, from your working muscles to the heart, brain, and other vital organs. Sometimes if a person just stops exercising after a workout, the blood will pool or stay in the tissues of the legs. This can make the person light-headed because not enough oxygenated blood is getting to the brain. So, the cooldown should be a 3–5 minute progressive recovery at a light intensity. Gradually proceed from your energetic HIIT workout to a mild pace. For instance, if your HIIT workout was walking briskly, jogging, or running, you would progress to a leisurely walk to cooldown.

Finally, do some total body stretching exercises to facilitate a full relaxation of your body and mind. Yes—mind. The stretches provide some mindful relaxation as you transition mentally from your workout to the next phase of your day.

To help you, I'll share my five favorite post-workout stretches along with instructions and pictures. I encourage you to do these stretches on an exercise mat.

CALF AND ACHILLES STRETCH

THE STRETCH ACTION: Stand in a lunge position with your toes facing forward. To stretch the calf, bend your front leg and keep your back leg straight. To add the Achilles tendon and soleus muscle stretch, bend the back leg slightly, keeping the heel on the floor. Hold each stretch for 15–30 seconds. Make sure you do both sides.

PERFORMANCE TIP: For steadiness, sometimes it is helpful to do these stretches with your hands placed against a wall or other immovable object.

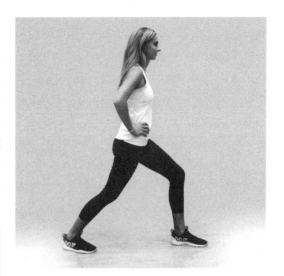

HALF-STRADDLE STRETCH

THE STRETCH ACTION: In a seated position, with one leg straight and the other leg bent, reach your chest forward toward the straight leg and hold for 15–30 seconds. Do this with both legs.

PERFORMANCE TIP: Keep your back straight and breathe slowly.

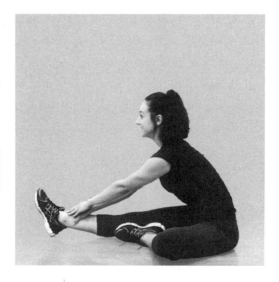

QUADRICEPS AND HIP FLEXORS

THE STRETCH ACTION: While lying on your side, grab below the knee and stretch the leg back. Hold this for 15–30 seconds and then repeat it on your other side.

> **PERFORMANCE TIP:** Focus on bringing the leg back so you feel a stretch in the top front of your thigh.

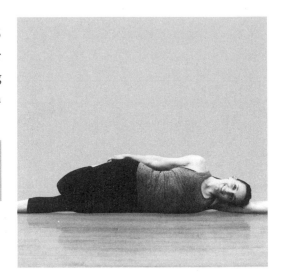

LOWER BACK STRETCH

THE STRETCH ACTION: While lying on your back, grab behind the knees and pull your legs toward your chest. Your legs should be extended with a slight bend. Hold this for 15–30 seconds.

> **PERFORMANCE TIP:** Try to keep your buttocks from rolling up off the floor.

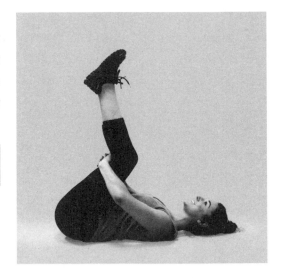

ABDOMINAL AND CHEST STRETCH

THE STRETCH ACTION: From a prone position, lift the shoulders and chest off the ground and support the upper torso with the elbows. Hold this for 15–30 seconds.

PERFORMANCE TIP: For a stretch with a greater range of motion, complete the same movement with your arms extended.

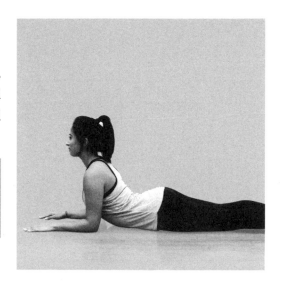

How Hard Should I Exercise?

TO REVIEW: HIIT WORKOUTS ARE A METHOD OF TRAINING THAT INVOLVES BOUTS OF high-intensity exercise (the WORK interval) followed by light-intensity RECOVERY periods of exercise, repeated at varying lengths of time. Recall also that the WORK intervals should be at an intensity that's comfortable but challenging, or comfortable but more challenging. Consequently, to maximize the success of this approach you are going to monitor both the WORK intervals and RECOVERY intervals. There are a number of ways to monitor exercise intensity scientifically, but to make things as effortless as possible, we will go over two equipment-free but accurate intensity-monitoring approaches you can rely on instead.

PRESENTING THE PERCEIVED EXERTION METHOD

The first approach I'd like you to use to assess the intensity of your HIIT workouts is the "perceived exertion" gauge. (You may recognize this from the very first pages of the book, where it was briefly discussed.) The concept of perceived exertion was originally introduced by Dr. Gunnar Borg in 1982 in the journal *Medicine & Science in Sports & Exercise*. With perceived exertion, you subjectively interpret various body sensations, such as heart rate, muscle and joint sensations, breathing intensity, and body temperature, to estimate your exercise intensity. Though at first it may seem imprecise, this technique has been validated by the research and found to be a particularly accurate way to monitor and assess your intensity.

I want everyone to be able to enjoy HIIT workouts, and the ease of this approach ensures that every person can enjoy HIIT workouts at their own personal pace. Exercise is for everyone—particularly when you do it at a personalized intensity level. As you continue your training, this same perceived exertion approach will work for you as you get more fit. That's because it's individualized: as part of the approach, you are always monitoring and modifying your workout depending on how you feel the day of your workout. So it's completely tailored toward *you*.

There are various perceived exertion scales, but for our purposes we'll rely on a scale between 0 and 10. For the high-intensity (WORK) interval of your HIIT workouts, I want you to strive for levels 5 or 6. At levels 5 and 6, the intensity should feel comfortable but challenging or comfortable but more challenging. For the RECOVERY interval of your HIIT workouts, try to attain a level between 2 and 4 on the scale. Choose light movement, mild-intensity exercise, or somewhat hard exercise during your RECOVERY interval. I always encourage students to monitor and adjust their WORK *and* RECOVERY intensity during their workouts. In my own workouts, when I start to fatigue, I decrease both my WORK and RECOVERY interval intensities as I head toward completion of the workout; I encourage you to do the same thing. For brevity's sake, let's use the acronym "PEI" for "perceived exertion intensity."

PERCEIVED EXERTION INTENSITY (PEI) SCALE

PEI	SUBJECTIVE LEVEL OF INTENSITY
0	No Exertion: Sitting quietly
1	Very light movement: Standing and strolling
2	Light movement: Normal walking pace
3	Mild intensity exercise: Brisk walking pace
4	Somewhat hard exercise: A good target intensity for moderate intensity, steady state exercise
5	Comfortable but challenging
6	Comfortable but more challenging
7	Exercise that is difficult to sustain
8	Demanding exercise you cannot sustain
9	Near maximal intensity exercise
10	All-out effort intensity

THE TALK TEST IS AN ACCURATE GAUGE OF EXERCISE INTENSITY, TOO!

In addition to PEI, the talk test is a very easy and accurate way to know if you are at the optimal HIIT training intensity level for your workouts. During your high-intensity interval, if you can speak any thirty-word phrase, such as the Pledge of Allegiance, or tell a short story, or carry on a conversation for about 30 seconds with moderate difficulty, you are right at the desired target for your WORK intervals. If you can't get through the thirty-word phrase, short story, or conversation, you are exercising too hard. During the RECOVERY intervals, you should be able to recite any 30-word phrase, tell a short story, or carry a conversation for 30 seconds with mild to no difficulty. Like the perceived exertion gauge, using a talk test to measure your level of effort may seem imprecise or inaccurate, but research has validated this simple test as an accurate way to interpret exercise intensity. It is totally individualized to how you feel during your workout—which is why we use it! It really works.

OVEREXERTION CAUTION!

It's appropriate to conclude a chapter on how hard you should exercise by briefly discussing the concept of overexertion. Sometimes, in the zeal to meet their fitness goals—or perhaps to keep up with a training partner—people will do too much during their workouts. This overexertion may trigger an unfamiliar feeling. When you're exercising, if you start to feel breathless, dizzy, tightness or pain in the chest, a loss of muscle control, or nausea, please stop what you are doing *immediately*. Your body is alerting you that something may be wrong with your present health condition. If you experience any of these symptoms, see your physician to determine the cause before doing any more workouts.

CHAPTER 19

Your HIIT Workouts Plan

I'D LIKE TO GO OVER A FEW DETAILS TO ENSURE THAT UNDERSTANDING THE HIIT WORKOUT designs is as effortless as possible. The title of each HIIT workout indicates its WORK/ RECOVERY ratio and whether it's in seconds, minutes, or a combination of both. To get a better understanding of what I mean, let's analyze the title of an actual workout: Workout #5: 30s/30s HIIT. First, as you can probably figure out, this is the fifth workout in the book. Next, the "30s/30s" alerts you right away that the WORK interval of this exercise is 30 seconds and the RECOVERY interval is 30 seconds. If you see "3m/3m" in the workout title, it tells you the WORK interval is 3 minutes and the RECOVERY interval is 3 minutes. Basically, the title of each HIIT workout prepares you for the workout itself.

Below the title of each workout I have crafted a workout blueprint for you to follow. As you'll notice, most of the HIIT workouts actually let you choose up to three workout lengths, each falling between 10 and 20 minutes in duration (not counting the warm-up and cooldown). So, counting the warm-up, cooldown, and workout, every workout in this book is about 30 minutes or less.

If you're wondering why they're short, here's why: the number one reason people state they do not workout is a lack of time. Simply put, most people say they just don't have enough time to fit exercise into their busy schedule. The great news is HIIT training has been shown in research to be a remarkably time-efficient type of training. In fact, a 2017 study in the *Journal of Diabetes Research* showed that participants doing HIIT attained the same body composition and cardiorespiratory benefits as people doing steady-state exercise, but in half the time. That's astounding! That's why all the workouts in *HIIT Your Limit* are 30 minutes or less.

That said, I welcome you to vary the length of each workout depending on how you feel. In each workout I suggest appropriate intensities for the high-intensity WORK intervals as well as the light-intensity RECOVERY intervals, using the perceived exertion and talk test gauges. On any day, and at any moment, feel empowered to modify the workout to best meet your desired level of exertion and duration. *You are in charge of every workout!*

For those of you doing swimming HIIT workouts, I suggest you do 2 laps at a comfortable-but-challenging intensity and time yourself. This will give you a time frame to work from when doing the HIIT WORK intervals. Do the same thing for your RECOVERY intervals: time yourself on 2 laps at a light to somewhat hard swimming intensity. You can't easily take a timer in the water with you, but you can gauge how many laps you do. Swimmers do this all the time.

Special surprise! With each workout I will also give you a motivational message, and I will conclude each workout with an exercise training tip. I have done this for many years in my fitness classes. It's my hope that you enjoy these moving messages and training tips as much as my students do.

HOW TO INTEGRATE HIIT WORKOUTS WITH YOUR STEADY-STATE WORKOUTS

Before we move on to the workouts, let's quickly review the American College of Sports Medicine (ACSM) guidelines for exercise. ACSM is the leading sports medicine organization in the world. In its exercise guidelines, ACSM encourages all adults to do at least 150 minutes of moderate-intensity exercise per week. Multiple shorter sessions of at least 10 minutes are acceptable for meeting this goal too.

With these guidelines in mind, I'd like to suggest you start with just two HIIT workouts a week. And, in order to ensure that you progress at a sustainable pace, you should begin with the shorter of the three workout options, the 10-minute workout. Let the rest of your 150 exercise minutes throughout the week be steady-state exercise.

Earlier in the book we defined steady-state exercise as continuous moderate-intensity aerobic workouts. Wow—that's a mouthful, so let's break it down. Steady-state exercise is when you exercise at the same intensity during the whole workout. Most people perform steady-state exercise at a somewhat hard intensity. Here's a common example: a 30-minute riding session on a stationary bike. Perform your steady-state workouts at an intensity level of 4, which is a somewhat hard intensity on the perceived exertion scale. As you get stronger from doing your workouts consistently, you can adapt the length of your HIIT workout, progressing from a 10-minute workout to a 15-minute workout and, eventually, a 20-minute one.

I invite you to try a different routine every time you do a HIIT workout, or stick with one for a short time and then progress to another. You should do at least two HIIT workouts a week and if over the course of a few weeks, you feel ready to exert yourself more, add a third HIIT workout day during the week. Once again, I suggest you start the third HIIT workout day with a 10-minute workout duration. When you add the third HIIT workout day, make sure you allow at least 48 hours between HIIT workouts. Eventually—when you're ready—you can take yourself up to four HIIT workouts a week, each separated by at least 24 hours, with the remainder of your exercise time dedicated to other steady-state cardiorespiratory workouts. Since everyone has a different fitness level and health status, I encourage you to individualize your workout progression. The take-away message is to progress gradually with your HIIT workouts, integrating them with your steady-state workouts as they fit your schedule best. You can do it! Also, at the end of the book I have provided you with a workout schedule to track your workouts. Please use this as it will help you see how much you improve as you progress with your exercise program.

You know what to do. Now let's HIIT it!

CHAPTER 20

Your HIIT Workouts—Enjoy!

WORKOUT #1: 60S/90S HIIT

MOTIVATIONAL MESSAGE: Every day, in every way, you're getting fitter and healthier.

TIMER SETTING: Set your timer to cue you ALTERNATELY at 60 seconds and 90 seconds.

EXERCISE MODE: Can be completed while walking, jogging, running, biking, elliptical striding, swimming, rowing, stair stepping, and/or using any type of cardio machine.

WARM-UP: Complete a 5–7 minute progressive warm-up at a perceived exertion intensity (PEI) level of 2–3 (light to mild-feeling intensity). Do the same exercise you will do for your HIIT workout.

HIIT WORKOUT DESIGN

	INTERVAL	DURATION	INTENSITY
BOUT 1	WORK Interval 1	60 seconds	PEI: Level 5: Feels challenging TALK Test: Moderate difficulty talking
	RECOVERY Interval 1	90 seconds	PEI: Level 2–4: Light movement to somewhat hard TALK Test: Mild to no difficulty talking
BOUT 2	WORK Interval 2	60 seconds	PEI: Level 5–6: Feels challenging to more challenging TALK Test: Moderate difficulty talking
	RECOVERY Interval 2	90 seconds	PEI: Level 2–4: Light movement to somewhat hard TALK Test: Mild to no difficulty talking

CHOOSE THE LENGTH OF THIS WORKOUT DEPENDING ON HOW YOU FEEL!

PROGRESSION: Start off with the 10-minute workout.

- For a 10-minute workout complete 4 BOUTS
- For a 15-minute workout complete 6 BOUTS
- For a 20-minute workout complete 8 BOUTS

COOLDOWN: 3–5 minute progressive recovery at a mild intensity

DO YOUR 5 STRETCHES: Calf and Achilles Stretch, Half-Straddle Stretch, Quadriceps and Hip Flexors, Lower Back Stretch, Abdominal and Chest Stretch

> **EXERCISE TIP:** Do not let the early awkwardness of doing HIIT workouts slow you down. Everyone has some growing pains. Also, try not to compare yourselves to others—you are in this training program for YOU.

WORKOUT #2: 60S/60S HIIT

MOTIVATIONAL MESSAGE: It's not what you want to do that counts, it's what you do.

TIMER SETTING: Set your timer to cue you every 60 seconds.

EXERCISE MODE: Can be completed while walking, jogging, running, biking, elliptical striding, swimming, rowing, stair stepping, and/or using any type of cardio machine.

WARM-UP: Complete a 5–7 minute progressive warm-up at a perceived exertion intensity (PEI) level of 2–3 (light to a mild-feeling intensity). Do the same exercise you will do for your HIIT workout.

HIIT WORKOUT DESIGN

	INTERVAL	DURATION	INTENSITY
BOUT 1	WORK Interval 1	60 seconds	PEI: Level 5: Feels challenging TALK Test: Moderate difficulty talking
	RECOVERY Interval 1	60 seconds	PEI: Level 2–4: Light movement to somewhat hard TALK Test: Mild to no difficulty talking

	INTERVAL	DURATION	INTENSITY
BOUT 2	WORK Interval 2	60 seconds	PEI: Level 5–6: Feels challenging to more challenging TALK Test: Moderate difficulty talking
	RECOVERY Interval 2	60 seconds	PEI: Level 2–4: Light movement to somewhat hard TALK Test: Mild to no difficulty talking

CHOOSE THE LENGTH OF THIS WORKOUT DEPENDING ON HOW YOU FEEL!

PROGRESSION: Start off with the 10-minute workout.

- For a 10-minute workout complete 5 BOUTS
- For a 15-minute workout complete 7 BOUTS
- For a 20-minute workout complete 10 BOUTS

COOLDOWN: 3–5 minute progressive recovery at a mild intensity

DO YOUR 5 STRETCHES: Calf and Achilles Stretch, Half-Straddle Stretch, Quadriceps and Hip Flexors, Lower Back Stretch, Abdominal and Chest Stretch

> **EXERCISE TIP:** Sometimes new HIIT exercisers will breathe erratically, shallowly, and/or ineffectively as they complete their initial HIIT workouts. Focus on the intervals and your subjective intensity, and let your breathing adjust to the workout. Try not to force yourself into a breathing pattern; the body will do this automatically.

WORKOUT #3: 60S/30S HIIT

MOTIVATIONAL MESSAGE: It's not the will to win, it's the will to prepare that builds the champion within you.

TIMER SETTING: Set your timer to cue you ALTERNATELY at 60 seconds and 30 seconds.

EXERCISE MODE: Can be completed while walking, jogging, running, biking, elliptical striding, swimming, rowing, stair stepping, and/or using any type of cardio machine.

WARM-UP: Complete a 5–7 progressive minute warm-up at a perceived exertion intensity (PEI) of 2–3 (light to mild-feeling intensity). Do the same exercise you will do for your HIIT workout.

HIIT WORKOUT DESIGN

	INTERVAL	DURATION	INTENSITY
BOUT 1	WORK Interval 1	60 seconds	PEI: Level 5: Feels challenging TALK Test: Moderate difficulty talking
	RECOVERY Interval 1	30 seconds	PEI: Level 2–4: Light movement to somewhat hard TALK Test: Mild to no difficulty talking
BOUT 2	WORK Interval 2	60 seconds	PEI: Level 5–6: Feels challenging to more challenging TALK Test: Moderate difficulty talking
	RECOVERY Interval 2	30 seconds	PEI: Level 2–4: Light movement to somewhat hard TALK Test: Mild to no difficulty talking

CHOOSE THE LENGTH OF THIS WORKOUT DEPENDING ON HOW YOU FEEL!

PROGRESSION: Start off with the 10-minute workout.

- For a 10-minute workout complete 6 BOUTS
- For a 15-minute workout complete 10 BOUTS
- For a 20-minute workout complete 13 BOUTS

COOLDOWN: 3–5 minute progressive recovery at a mild intensity

DO YOUR 5 STRETCHES: Calf and Achilles Stretch, Half-Straddle Stretch, Quadriceps and Hip Flexors, Lower Back Stretch, Abdominal and Chest Stretch

EXERCISE TIP: You do not need to consume any additional salt after your workout. There is plenty of salt from the food you eat and what you sprinkle on your meals. Excess salt can irritate the stomach, dry out body tissues, and raise your blood pressure.

WORKOUT #4: 90S/30S HIIT

MOTIVATIONAL MESSAGE: You are eating healthier and healthier, each and every day.

TIMER SETTING: Set your timer to cue you ALTERNATELY at 90 seconds and 30 seconds.

EXERCISE MODE: Can be completed while walking, jogging, running, biking, elliptical striding, swimming, rowing, stair stepping, and/or using any type of cardio machine.

WARM-UP: Complete a 5–7 minute progressive warm-up at a perceived exertion intensity (PEI) of 2–3 (light to mild-feeling intensity). Do the same exercise you will do for your HIIT workout.

HIIT WORKOUT DESIGN

	INTERVAL	DURATION	INTENSITY
BOUT 1	WORK Interval 1	90 seconds	PEI: Level 5: Feels challenging TALK Test: Moderate difficulty talking
BOUT 1	RECOVERY Interval 1	30 seconds	PEI: Level 2–4: Light movement to somewhat hard TALK Test: Mild to no difficulty talking
BOUT 2	WORK Interval 2	90 seconds	PEI: Level 5–6: Feels challenging to more challenging TALK Test: Moderate difficulty talking
BOUT 2	RECOVERY Interval 2	30 seconds	PEI: Level 2–4: Light movement to somewhat hard TALK Test: Mild to no difficulty talking

CHOOSE THE LENGTH OF THIS WORKOUT DEPENDING ON HOW YOU FEEL!

PROGRESSION: Start off with the 10-minute workout.

- For a 10-minute workout complete 5 BOUTS
- For a 15-minute workout complete 7 BOUTS
- For a 20-minute workout complete 10 BOUTS

COOLDOWN: 3–5 minute progressive recovery at a mild intensity

DO YOUR 5 STRETCHES: Calf and Achilles Stretch, Half-Straddle Stretch, Quadriceps and Hip Flexors, Lower Back Stretch, Abdominal and Chest Stretch

> **EXERCISE TIP:** Laser focus on attaining the perceived exertion training intensities for your WORK and RECOVERY intervals. However, as you fatigue, lessen the intensity to complete your workouts.

WORKOUT #5: 30S/30S HIIT

MOTIVATIONAL MESSAGE: Every workout you do is a priceless gift to your personal health.

TIMER SETTING: Set your timer to cue you ALTERNATELY every 30 seconds.

EXERCISE MODE: Can be completed while walking, jogging, running, biking, elliptical striding, swimming, rowing, stair stepping, and/or using any type of cardio machine.

WARM-UP: Complete a 5–7 minute progressive warm-up at a perceived exertion intensity (PEI) of 2–3 (light to mild-feeling intensity). Do the same exercise you will do for your HIIT workout.

HIIT WORKOUT DESIGN

	INTERVAL	DURATION	INTENSITY
BOUT 1	WORK Interval 1	30 seconds	PEI: Level 5: Feels challenging TALK Test: Moderate difficulty talking
BOUT 1	RECOVERY Interval 1	30 seconds	PEI: Level 2–4: Light movement to somewhat hard TALK Test: Mild to no difficulty talking
BOUT 2	WORK Interval 2	30 seconds	PEI: Level 5–6: Feels challenging to more challenging TALK Test: Moderate difficulty talking
BOUT 2	RECOVERY Interval 2	30 seconds	PEI: Level 2–4: Light movement to somewhat hard TALK Test: Mild to no difficulty talking

CHOOSE THE LENGTH OF THIS WORKOUT DEPENDING ON HOW YOU FEEL!

PROGRESSION: Start off with the 10-minute workout.

- For a 10-minute workout complete 10 BOUTS
- For a 15-minute workout complete 15 BOUTS
- For a 20-minute workout complete 20 BOUTS

COOLDOWN: 3–5 minute progressive recovery at a mild intensity

DO YOUR 5 STRETCHES: Calf and Achilles Stretch, Half-Straddle Stretch, Quadriceps and Hip Flexors, Lower Back Stretch, Abdominal and Chest Stretch

EXERCISE TIP: Try to multi-mode your HIIT workouts. Multi-mode training is an exercise method in which you complete your HIIT workouts in different exercise modes. For instance, one day you complete your HIIT workout on a treadmill and another day you do your workout on a bike. Keep changing the modes of your exercise, depending on what is accessible to you. The use of multi-mode training will prevent you from getting bored with your workouts, and may also help prevent overtraining injuries.

WORKOUT #6: 30S/45S HIIT

MOTIVATIONAL MESSAGE: The power is within you to succeed. Take charge of your health, fitness, and quality of life.

TIMER SETTING: Set your timer to cue you ALTERNATELY at 30 seconds and 45 seconds

EXERCISE MODE: Can be completed while walking, jogging, running, biking, elliptical striding, swimming, rowing, stair stepping, and/or using any type of cardio machine.

WARM-UP: Complete a 5–7 minute progressive warm-up at a perceived exertion intensity (PEI) of 2–3 (light to mild-feeling intensity). Do the same exercise you will do for your HIIT workout.

HIIT WORKOUT DESIGN

	INTERVAL	DURATION	INTENSITY
BOUT 1	WORK Interval 1	30 seconds	PEI: Level 5: Feels challenging TALK Test: Moderate difficulty talking
	RECOVERY Interval 1	45 seconds	PEI: Level 2–4: Light movement to somewhat hard TALK Test: Mild to no difficulty talking
BOUT 2	WORK Interval 2	30 seconds	PEI: Level 5–6: Feels challenging to more challenging TALK Test: Moderate difficulty talking
	RECOVERY Interval 2	45 seconds	PEI: Level 2–4: Light movement to somewhat hard TALK Test: Mild to no difficulty talking

CHOOSE THE LENGTH OF THIS WORKOUT DEPENDING ON HOW YOU FEEL!

PROGRESSION: Start off with the 10-minute workout.

- For a 10-minute workout complete 8 BOUTS
- For a 15-minute workout complete 12 BOUTS
- For a 20-minute workout complete 16 BOUTS

COOLDOWN: 3–5 minute progressive recovery at a mild intensity

DO YOUR 5 STRETCHES: Calf and Achilles Stretch, Half-Straddle Stretch, Quadriceps and Hip Flexors, Lower Back Stretch, Abdominal and Chest Stretch

EXERCISE TIP: Regular exercise improves your mental well-being. Some psychological benefits include improvements in self-confidence, increased alertness, clearer thinking, positive coping, and optimistic mood changes.

WORKOUT #7: 30S/60S HIIT

MOTIVATIONAL MESSAGE: Every workout counts; make the most of each one.

TIMER SETTING: Set your timer to cue you ALTERNATELY at 30 seconds and 60 seconds

EXERCISE MODE: Can be completed while walking, jogging, running, biking, elliptical striding, swimming, rowing, stair stepping, and/or using any type of cardio machine.

WARM-UP: Complete a 5–7 minute progressive warm-up at a perceived exertion intensity (PEI) of 2–3 (light to mild-feeling intensity). Do the same exercise you will do for your HIIT workout.

HIIT WORKOUT DESIGN

	INTERVAL	DURATION	INTENSITY
BOUT 1	WORK Interval 1	30 seconds	PEI: Level 5: Feels challenging TALK Test: Moderate difficulty talking
	RECOVERY Interval 1	60 seconds	PEI: Level 2–4: Light movement to somewhat hard TALK Test: Mild to no difficulty talking
BOUT 2	WORK Interval 2	30 seconds	PEI: Level 5–6: Feels challenging to more challenging TALK Test: Moderate difficulty talking
	RECOVERY Interval 2	60 seconds	PEI: Level 2–4: Light movement to somewhat hard TALK Test: Mild to no difficulty talking

CHOOSE THE LENGTH OF THIS WORKOUT DEPENDING ON HOW YOU FEEL!

PROGRESSION: Start off with the 10-minute workout.

- For a 10-minute workout complete 7 BOUTS
- For a 15-minute workout complete 10 BOUTS
- For a 20-minute workout complete 13 BOUTS

COOLDOWN: 3–5 minute progressive recovery at a mild intensity

DO YOUR 5 STRETCHES: Calf and Achilles Stretch, Half-Straddle Stretch, Quadriceps and Hip Flexors, Lower Back Stretch, Abdominal and Chest Stretch

EXERCISE TIP: For newcomers, exercise can feel like a difficult behavior to learn. Research shows it takes about 6 months to become hooked on exercise as a way of life.

WORKOUT #8: 30S/90S HIIT

MOTIVATIONAL MESSAGE: On some days you need to tell yourself: get out there and do your workout. After your workout is completed, you will feel very empowered.

TIMER SETTING: Set your timer to cue you ALTERNATELY at 30 seconds and 90 seconds.

EXERCISE MODE: Can be completed while walking, jogging, running, biking, elliptical striding, swimming, rowing, stair stepping, and/or using any type of cardio machine.

WARM-UP: Complete a 5–7 minute progressive warm-up at a perceived exertion intensity (PEI) level of 2–3 (light to mild-feeling intensity). Do the same exercise you will do for your HIIT workout.

HIIT WORKOUT DESIGN

	INTERVAL	DURATION	INTENSITY
BOUT 1	WORK Interval 1	30 seconds	PEI: Level 5: Feels challenging TALK Test: Moderate difficulty talking
BOUT 1	RECOVERY Interval 1	90 seconds	PEI: Level 2–4: Light movement to somewhat hard TALK Test: Mild to no difficulty talking
BOUT 2	WORK Interval 2	30 seconds	PEI: Level 5–6: Feels challenging to more challenging TALK Test: Moderate difficulty talking
BOUT 2	RECOVERY Interval 2	90 seconds	PEI: Level 2–4: Light movement to somewhat hard TALK Test: Mild to no difficulty talking

CHOOSE THE LENGTH OF THIS WORKOUT DEPENDING ON HOW YOU FEEL!

PROGRESSION: Start off with the 10-minute workout.

- For a 10-minute workout complete 5 BOUTS
- For a 15-minute workout complete 7 BOUTS
- For a 20-minute workout complete 10 BOUTS

COOLDOWN: 3–5 minute progressive recovery at a mild intensity

DO YOUR 5 STRETCHES: Calf and Achilles Stretch, Half-Straddle Stretch, Quadriceps and Hip Flexors, Lower Back Stretch, Abdominal and Chest Stretch

EXERCISE TIP: Exercise slows down the body's physiological deterioration. This gives you a better quality of life and more energy as you age.

WORKOUT #9: 3M/3M HIIT

MOTIVATIONAL MESSAGE: With each workout completed, you are overcoming doubts about exercise as a way of life for you.

TIMER SETTING: Set your timer to cue you every 3 minutes.

EXERCISE MODE: Can be completed while walking, jogging, running, biking, elliptical striding, swimming, rowing, stair stepping, and/or using any type of cardio machine.

WARM-UP: Complete a 5–7 minute progressive warm-up at a perceived exertion intensity (PEI) level of 2–3 (light to mild-feeling intensity). Do the same exercise you will do for your HIIT workout.

HIIT WORKOUT DESIGN

	INTERVAL	DURATION	INTENSITY
BOUT 1	WORK Interval 1	3 minutes	PEI: Level 5: Feels challenging TALK Test: Moderate difficulty talking
BOUT 1	RECOVERY Interval 1	3 minutes	PEI: Level 2–4: Light movement to somewhat hard TALK Test: Mild to no difficulty talking
BOUT 2	WORK Interval 2	3 minutes	PEI: Level 5–6: Feels challenging to more challenging TALK Test: Moderate difficulty talking
BOUT 2	RECOVERY Interval 2	3 minutes	PEI: Level 2–4: Light movement to somewhat hard TALK Test: Mild to no difficulty talking

CHOOSE THE LENGTH OF THIS WORKOUT DEPENDING ON HOW YOU FEEL!

PROGRESSION: Start off with the 12-minute workout.
- For a 12-minute workout complete 2 BOUTS
- For an 18-minute workout complete 3 BOUTS

COOLDOWN: 3–5 minute progressive recovery at a mild intensity

DO YOUR 5 STRETCHES: Calf and Achilles Stretch, Half-Straddle Stretch, Quadriceps and Hip Flexors, Lower Back Stretch, Abdominal and Chest Stretch

EXERCISE TIP: Keep your HIIT workouts a little lighter in hot, humid environments, where sweat does not evaporate as well to cool you off.

WORKOUT #10: 3M/4M HIIT

MOTIVATIONAL MESSAGE: The road to health, fitness, and happiness has no finish line.

TIMER SETTING: Set your timer to cue you ALTERNATELY at 3 minutes and 4 minutes.

EXERCISE MODE: Can be completed while walking, jogging, running, biking, elliptical striding, swimming, rowing, stair stepping, and/or using any type of cardio machine.

WARM-UP: Complete a 5–7 minute progressive warm-up at a perceived exertion intensity (PEI) level of 2–3 (light to mild-feeling intensity). Do the same exercise you will do for your HIIT workout.

HIIT WORKOUT DESIGN

	INTERVAL	DURATION	INTENSITY
BOUT 1	WORK Interval 1	3 minutes	PEI: Level 5: Feels challenging TALK Test: Moderate difficulty talking
	RECOVERY Interval 1	4 minutes	PEI: Level 2–4: Light movement to somewhat hard TALK Test: Mild to no difficulty talking
BOUT 2	WORK Interval 2	3 minutes	PEI: Level 5–6: Feels challenging to more challenging TALK Test: Moderate difficulty talking
	RECOVERY Interval 2	4 minutes	PEI: Level 2–4: Light movement to somewhat hard TALK Test: Mild to no difficulty talking

CHOOSE THE LENGTH OF THIS WORKOUT DEPENDING ON HOW YOU FEEL!

PROGRESSION: Start off with the 14-minute workout.

- For a 14-minute workout complete 2 BOUTS
- For a 21-minute workout complete 3 BOUTS

COOLDOWN: 3–5 minute progressive recovery at a mild intensity

DO YOUR 5 STRETCHES: Calf and Achilles Stretch, Half-Straddle Stretch, Quadriceps and Hip Flexors, Lower Back Stretch, Abdominal and Chest Stretch

> **EXERCISE TIP:** When doing your stretches at the end of the workout, allow yourself to breathe slowly and let the exhalation be about 1.5 times longer than the inhalation. When you exhale, there is a total relaxation of your respiratory muscles, which facilitates a total relaxation of mind and body.

WORKOUT #11: 3M/6M HIIT

MOTIVATIONAL MESSAGE: The best way to work out procrastination is to work through it, mentally and physically.

TIMER SETTING: Set your timer to cue you ALTERNATELY at 3 minutes and 6 minutes.

EXERCISE MODE: Can be completed while walking, jogging, running, biking, elliptical striding, swimming, rowing, stair stepping, and/or using any type of cardio machine.

WARM-UP: Complete a 5–7 progressive minute warm-up at a perceived exertion intensity (PEI) level of 2–3 (light to mild-feeling intensity). Do the same exercise you will do for your HIIT workout.

HIIT WORKOUT DESIGN

	INTERVAL	DURATION	INTENSITY
BOUT 1	WORK Interval 1	3 minutes	PEI: Level 5: Feels challenging TALK Test: Moderate difficulty talking
BOUT 1	RECOVERY Interval 1	6 minutes	PEI: Level 2–4: Light movement to somewhat hard TALK Test: Mild to no difficulty talking
BOUT 2	WORK Interval 2	3 minutes	PEI: Level 5–6: Feels challenging to more challenging TALK Test: Moderate difficulty talking
BOUT 2	RECOVERY Interval 2	6 minutes	PEI: Level 2–4: Light movement to somewhat hard TALK Test: Mild to no difficulty talking

CHOOSE THE LENGTH OF THIS WORKOUT DEPENDING ON HOW YOU FEEL!

PROGRESSION: Start off with the 9-minute workout.

- For a 9-minute workout complete 1 BOUT
- For an 18-minute workout complete 2 BOUTS

COOLDOWN: 3–5 minute progressive recovery at a mild intensity

DO YOUR 5 STRETCHES: Calf and Achilles Stretch, Half-Straddle Stretch, Quadriceps and Hip Flexors, Lower Back Stretch, Abdominal and Chest Stretch

EXERCISE TIP: Some people think doing fast, twisting movements with their waist will help narrow it. This is an exercise myth. These movements put shear stress on the spine and should be avoided.

WORKOUT #12: 4M/3M HIIT

MOTIVATIONAL MESSAGE: Every workout leads to a treasure trove of positive changes in your body.

TIMER SETTING: Set your timer to cue you ALTERNATELY at 4 minutes and 3 minutes.

EXERCISE MODE: Can be completed while walking, jogging, running, biking, elliptical striding, swimming, rowing, stair stepping, and/or using any type of cardio machine.

WARM-UP: Complete a 5–7 minute progressive warm-up at a perceived exertion intensity (PEI) of 2–3 (light to mild-feeling intensity). Do the same exercise you will do for your HIIT workout.

HIIT WORKOUT DESIGN

	INTERVAL	DURATION	INTENSITY
BOUT 1	WORK Interval 1	4 minutes	PEI: Level 5: Feels challenging TALK Test: Moderate difficulty talking
	RECOVERY Interval 1	3 minutes	PEI: Level 2–4: Light movement to somewhat hard TALK Test: Mild to no difficulty talking
BOUT 2	WORK Interval 2	4 minutes	PEI: Level 5–6: Feels challenging to more challenging TALK Test: Moderate difficulty talking
	RECOVERY Interval 2	3 minutes	PEI: Level 2–4: Light movement to somewhat hard TALK Test: Mild to no difficulty talking

CHOOSE THE LENGTH OF THIS WORKOUT DEPENDING ON HOW YOU FEEL!

PROGRESSION: Start off with the 14-minute workout.

- For a 14-minute workout complete 2 BOUTS
- For a 21-minute workout complete 3 BOUTS

COOLDOWN: 3–5 minute progressive recovery at a mild intensity

DO YOUR 5 STRETCHES: Calf and Achilles Stretch, Half-Straddle Stretch, Quadriceps and Hip Flexors, Lower Back Stretch, Abdominal and Chest Stretch

> **EXERCISE TIP:** Take a yoga class periodically if you can fit it in your schedule. Yoga has been shown to increase flexibility, balance, posture, and muscular endurance. It may also help to reduce stress.

WORKOUT #13: 4M/2M HIIT

MOTIVATIONAL MESSAGE: When it comes to setting personal priorities, let your health be number 1.

TIMER SETTING: Set your timer to cue you ALTERNATELY at 4 minutes and 2 minutes.

EXERCISE MODE: Can be completed while walking, jogging, running, biking, elliptical striding, swimming, rowing, stair stepping, and/or using any type of cardio machine.

WARM-UP: Complete a 5–7 minute progressive warm-up at a perceived exertion intensity (PEI) level of 2–3 (light to mild-feeling intensity). Do the same exercise you will do for your HIIT workout.

HIIT WORKOUT DESIGN

	INTERVAL	DURATION	INTENSITY
BOUT 1	WORK Interval 1	4 minutes	PEI: Level 5: Feels challenging TALK Test: Moderate difficulty talking
BOUT 1	RECOVERY Interval 1	2 minutes	PEI: Level 2–4: Light movement to somewhat hard TALK Test: Mild to no difficulty talking
BOUT 2	WORK Interval 2	4 minutes	PEI: Level 5–6: Feels challenging to more challenging TALK Test: Moderate difficulty talking
BOUT 2	RECOVERY Interval 2	2 minutes	PEI: Level 2–4: Light movement to somewhat hard TALK Test: Mild to no difficulty talking

CHOOSE THE LENGTH OF THIS WORKOUT DEPENDING ON HOW YOU FEEL!

PROGRESSION: Start off with the 12-minute workout.

- For a 12-minute workout complete 2 BOUTS
- For an 18-minute workout complete 3 BOUTS

COOLDOWN: 3–5 minute progressive recovery at a mild intensity

DO YOUR 5 STRETCHES: Calf and Achilles Stretch, Half-Straddle Stretch, Quadriceps and Hip Flexors, Lower Back Stretch, Abdominal and Chest Stretch

EXERCISE TIP: Exercises performed incorrectly can lead to injury. Poor exercise technique is most likely to occur during the later stages of a workout, when you are becoming tired.

WORKOUT #14: 8S/12S HIIT

MOTIVATIONAL MESSAGE: If you can believe you will achieve your health and fitness goals, you will achieve them. Success starts in the mind.

TIMER SETTING: Set your timer to cue you ALTERNATELY at 8 seconds and 12 seconds

EXERCISE MODE: Because of the very fast interval times with this HIIT workout, I suggest you complete it while doing one of the following exercises only: walking or jogging on land (not a treadmill), biking, elliptical striding, rowing, or stair stepping.

WARM-UP: Complete a 5–7 minute progressive warm-up at a perceived exertion intensity (PEI) level of 2–3 (light to mild-feeling intensity). Do the same exercise you will do for your HIIT workout.

HIIT WORKOUT DESIGN

	INTERVAL	DURATION	INTENSITY
BOUT 1	WORK Interval 1	8 seconds	PEI: Level 5: Feels challenging TALK Test: Moderate difficulty talking
BOUT 1	RECOVERY Interval 1	12 seconds	PEI: Level 2–4: Light movement to somewhat hard TALK Test: Mild to no difficulty talking
BOUT 2	WORK Interval 2	8 seconds	PEI: Level 5–6: Feels challenging to more challenging TALK Test: Moderate difficulty talking
BOUT 2	RECOVERY Interval 2	12 seconds	PEI: Level 2–4: Light movement to somewhat hard TALK Test: Mild to no difficulty talking

CHOOSE THE LENGTH OF THIS WORKOUT DEPENDING ON HOW YOU FEEL!

PROGRESSION: Start off with the 10-minute workout.

- For a 10-minute workout complete 30 BOUTS
- For a 15-minute workout complete 45 BOUTS
- For a 20-minute workout complete 60 BOUTS

COOLDOWN: 3–5 minute progressive recovery at a mild intensity

DO YOUR 5 STRETCHES: Calf and Achilles Stretch, Half-Straddle Stretch, Quadriceps and Hip Flexors, Lower Back Stretch, Abdominal and Chest Stretch

EXERCISE TIP: After a workout some people like to bend over and stretch toward their toes. This may put too much stress on the spine. Instead, do the half-straddle stretch I have selected for you. It's safer and a better stretch for the muscles on the back of the thigh.

WORKOUT #15: 15S/15S HIIT

MOTIVATIONAL MESSAGE: Permit yourself to become a role model of healthy behaviors for your family and friends.

TIMER SETTING: Set your timer to cue you every 15 seconds.

EXERCISE MODE: Because of the very fast intervals times with this HIIT workout, I suggest you complete it while doing one of the following exercises only: walking or jogging on land (not a treadmill), biking, elliptical striding, rowing, and stair stepping.

WARM-UP: Complete a 5–7 minute progressive warm-up at a perceived exertion intensity (PEI) of 2–3 (light to mild-feeling intensity). Do the same exercise you will do for your HIIT workout.

HIIT WORKOUT DESIGN

	INTERVAL	DURATION	INTENSITY
BOUT 1	WORK Interval 1	15 seconds	PEI: Level 5: Feels challenging TALK Test: Moderate difficulty talking
	RECOVERY Interval 1	15 seconds	PEI: Level 2–4: Light movement to somewhat hard TALK Test: Mild to no difficulty talking
BOUT 2	WORK Interval 2	15 seconds	PEI: Level 5–6: Feels challenging to more challenging TALK Test: Moderate difficulty talking
	RECOVERY Interval 2	15 seconds	PEI: Level 2–4: Light movement to somewhat hard TALK Test: Mild to no difficulty talking

CHOOSE THE LENGTH OF THIS WORKOUT DEPENDING ON HOW YOU FEEL!

PROGRESSION: Start off with the 10-minute workout.

- For a 10-minute workout complete 20 BOUTS
- For a 15-minute workout complete 30 BOUTS
- For a 20-minute workout complete 40 BOUTS

COOLDOWN: 3–5 minute progressive recovery at a mild intensity

DO YOUR 5 STRETCHES: Calf and Achilles Stretch, Half-Straddle Stretch, Quadriceps and Hip Flexors, Lower Back Stretch, Abdominal and Chest Stretch

> **EXERCISE TIP:** If you're doing a biking HIIT workout on a stationary bike, make sure you have adequate ventilation to properly cool the body during the workout. If the workout environment is too hot your heart rate and blood pressure will elevate, putting undue stress on the heart.

WORKOUT #16: 30S/4.5M HIIT

MOTIVATIONAL MESSAGE: If you can learn from your lapses (dietary, fitness, health), you are on the way to preventing them from occurring again.

TIMER SETTING: Set your timer to cue you ALTERNATELY at 30 seconds and 4.5 minutes

EXERCISE MODE: Can be completed while walking, jogging, running, biking, elliptical striding, swimming, rowing, stair stepping, and/or using any type of cardio machine.

WARM-UP: Complete a 5–7 minute progressive warm-up at a perceived exertion intensity (PEI) level of 2–3 (light to mild-feeling intensity). Do the same exercise you will do for your HIIT workout.

HIIT WORKOUT DESIGN

	INTERVAL	DURATION	INTENSITY
BOUT 1	WORK Interval 1	30 seconds	PEI: Level 5: Feels challenging TALK Test: Moderate difficulty talking
BOUT 1	RECOVERY Interval 1	4.5 minutes	PEI: Level 2–4: Light movement to somewhat hard TALK Test: Mild to no difficulty talking
BOUT 2	WORK Interval 2	30 seconds	PEI: Level 5–6: Feels challenging to more challenging TALK Test: Moderate difficulty talking
BOUT 2	RECOVERY Interval 2	4.5 minutes	PEI: Level 2–4: Light movement to somewhat hard TALK Test: Mild to no difficulty talking

CHOOSE THE LENGTH OF THIS WORKOUT DEPENDING ON HOW YOU FEEL!

PROGRESSION: Start off with the 10-minute workout.

- For a 10-minute workout complete 2 BOUTS
- For a 15-minute workout complete 3 BOUTS
- For a 20-minute workout complete 4 BOUTS

COOLDOWN: 3–5 minute progressive recovery at a mild intensity

DO YOUR 5 STRETCHES: Calf and Achilles Stretch, Half-Straddle Stretch, Quadriceps and Hip Flexors, Lower Back Stretch, Abdominal and Chest Stretch

> **EXERCISE TIP:** Research shows the color green positively influences your workout intensity and exercise mood. If you have a park or exercise trail accessible, definitely try working out in a green environment for an enjoyable and better challenge.

WORKOUT #17: 4M/1-2-4M HIIT

MOTIVATIONAL MESSAGE: Exercise has many immediate and delayed benefits. Enjoy them all as they occur.

TIMER SETTING: I often just use a hand watch or clock on an exercise device for this workout. Note the bout durations below in the workout plan.

EXERCISE MODE: Can be completed while walking, jogging, running, biking, elliptical striding, swimming, rowing, stair stepping, and/or using any type of cardio machine.

WARM-UP: Complete a 5–7 minute progressive warm-up at a perceived exertion intensity (PEI) of 2–3 (light to mild-feeling intensity). Do the same exercise you will do for your HIIT workout.

HIIT WORKOUT DESIGN: This routine is referred to as a variable recovery HIIT routine, and it is a very unique HIIT workout. Pay special attention to how each recovery period varies in length. Please only do this HIIT routine one time through.

	INTERVAL	DURATION	INTENSITY
BOUT 1	WORK Interval 1	4 minutes	PEI: Level 5: Feels challenging TALK Test: Moderate difficulty talking
	RECOVERY Interval 1	1 minute	PEI: Level 2–4: Light movement to somewhat hard TALK Test: Mild to no difficulty talking

	INTERVAL	DURATION	INTENSITY
BOUT 2	WORK Interval 2	4 minutes	PEI: Level 5–6: Feels challenging to more challenging TALK Test: Moderate difficulty talking
	RECOVERY Interval 2	2 minutes	PEI: Level 2–4: Light movement to somewhat hard TALK Test: Mild to no difficulty talking
BOUT 3	WORK Interval 2	4 minutes	PEI: Level 5–6: Feels challenging to more challenging TALK Test: Moderate difficulty talking
	RECOVERY Interval 2	4 minutes	PEI: Level 2–4: Light movement to somewhat hard TALK Test: Mild to no difficulty talking

PROGRESSION: Complete all 3 bouts of this workout just once.

- For a 19-minute workout complete ALL BOUTS.

COOLDOWN: 3–5 minute progressive recovery at a mild intensity

DO YOUR 5 STRETCHES: Calf and Achilles Stretch, Half-Straddle Stretch, Quadriceps and Hip Flexors, Lower Back Stretch, Abdominal and Chest Stretch

> **EXERCISE TIP:** When it comes to health benefits, the research shows that exercise intensity is more important than exercise duration. I have specifically designed your workouts to be 30 minutes or less (including the warm-up and cooldown). As you progress, gradually challenge yourself a little more during the HIIT WORK intervals for greater health outcomes.

WORKOUT #18: 5M/5M HIIT

MOTIVATIONAL MESSAGE: Do not follow your passion—live your passion.

TIMER SETTING: Set your timer to cue you every 5 minutes.

EXERCISE MODE: Can be completed while walking, jogging, running, biking, elliptical striding, swimming, rowing, stair stepping, and/or using any type of cardio machine.

WARM-UP: Complete a 5–7 minute progressive warm-up at a perceived exertion intensity (PEI) level of 2–3 (light to mild-feeling intensity). Do the same exercise you will do for your HIIT workout.

HIIT WORKOUT DESIGN

	INTERVAL	DURATION	INTENSITY
BOUT 1	WORK Interval 1	5 minutes	PEI: Level 5: Feels challenging TALK Test: Moderate difficulty talking
	RECOVERY Interval 1	5 minutes	PEI: Level 2–4: Light movement to somewhat hard TALK Test: Mild to no difficulty talking
BOUT 2	WORK Interval 2	5 minutes	PEI: Level 5–6: Feels challenging to more challenging TALK Test: Moderate difficulty talking
	RECOVERY Interval 2	5 minutes	PEI: Level 2–4: Light movement to somewhat hard TALK Test: Mild to no difficulty talking

CHOOSE THE LENGTH OF THIS WORKOUT DEPENDING ON HOW YOU FEEL!

PROGRESSION: Start off with the 10-minute workout.

- For a 10-minute workout complete 1 BOUT
- For a 20-minute workout complete 2 BOUTS

COOLDOWN: 3–5 minute progressive recovery at a mild intensity

DO YOUR 5 STRETCHES: Calf and Achilles Stretch, Half-Straddle Stretch, Quadriceps and Hip Flexors, Lower Back Stretch, Abdominal and Chest Stretch

> **EXERCISE TIP:** Listening to upbeat music during a workout has been shown to enhance a person's workout intensity and duration. Create some stimulating playlists and try working out with them for some stirring workouts.

WORKOUT #19: 2M/2M HIIT

MOTIVATIONAL MESSAGE: Take charge of your life, and live for greatness.

TIMER SETTING: Set your timer to cue you ALTERNATELY at 2 minutes and 2 minutes.

EXERCISE MODE: Can be completed while walking, jogging, running, biking, elliptical striding, swimming, rowing, stair stepping, and/or using any type of cardio machine.

WARM-UP: Complete a 5–7 minute progressive warm-up at a perceived exertion intensity (PEI) level of 2–3 (light to mild-feeling). Do the same exercise you will do for your HIIT workout.

HIIT WORKOUT DESIGN

	INTERVAL	DURATION	INTENSITY
BOUT 1	WORK Interval 1	2 minutes	PEI: Level 5: Feels challenging TALK Test: Moderate difficulty talking
	RECOVERY Interval 1	2 minutes	PEI: Level 2–4: Light movement to somewhat hard TALK Test: Mild to no difficulty talking
BOUT 2	WORK Interval 2	2 minutes	PEI: Level 5–6: Feels challenging to more challenging TALK Test: Moderate difficulty talking
	RECOVERY Interval 2	2 minutes	PEI: Level 2–4: Light movement to somewhat hard TALK Test: Mild to no difficulty talking

CHOOSE THE LENGTH OF THIS WORKOUT DEPENDING ON HOW YOU FEEL!

PROGRESSION: Start off with the 8-minute workout.

- For a 12-minute workout complete 3 BOUTS
- For a 16-minute workout complete 4 BOUTS
- For a 20-minute workout complete 5 BOUTS

COOLDOWN: 3–5 minute progressive recovery at a mild intensity

DO YOUR 5 STRETCHES: Calf and Achilles Stretch, Half-Straddle Stretch, Quadriceps and Hip Flexors, Lower Back Stretch, Abdominal and Chest Stretch

EXERCISE TIP: Many people find it easier to adhere to an exercise schedule when they exercise in the morning, before beginning the many tasks and responsibilities of their day.

WORKOUT #20: 2M/1M HIIT

MOTIVATIONAL MESSAGE: To be your best at anything, do your best in everything you do.

TIMER SETTING: Set your timer to cue you ALTERNATELY at 2 minutes and 1 minute.

EXERCISE MODE: Can be completed while walking, jogging, running, biking, elliptical striding, swimming, rowing, stair stepping, and/or using any type of cardio machine.

WARM-UP: Complete a 5–7 progressive minute warm-up at a perceived exertion intensity (PEI) level of 2–3 (light to mild-feeling intensity). Do the same exercise you will do for your HIIT workout.

HIIT WORKOUT DESIGN

	INTERVAL	DURATION	INTENSITY
BOUT 1	WORK Interval 1	2 minutes	PEI: Level 5: Feels challenging TALK Test: Moderate difficulty talking
	RECOVERY Interval 1	1 minute	PEI: Level 2–4: Light movement to somewhat hard TALK Test: Mild to no difficulty talking
BOUT 2	WORK Interval 2	2 minutes	PEI: Level 5–6: Feels challenging to more challenging TALK Test: Moderate difficulty talking
	RECOVERY Interval 2	1 minute	PEI: Level 2–4: Light movement to somewhat hard TALK Test: Mild to no difficulty talking

CHOOSE THE LENGTH OF THIS WORKOUT DEPENDING ON HOW YOU FEEL!

PROGRESSION: Start off with the 9-minute workout.

- For a 9-minute workout complete 3 BOUTS

- For a 15-minute workout complete 5 BOUTS

- For a 21-minute workout complete 7 BOUTS

COOLDOWN: 3–5 minute progressive recovery at a mild intensity

DO YOUR 5 STRETCHES: Calf and Achilles Stretch, Half-Straddle Stretch, Quadriceps and Hip Flexors, Lower Back Stretch, Abdominal and Chest Stretch

> **EXERCISE TIP:** Definitely hydrate during all of your HIIT workouts, since sweating during your workouts depletes body water. Do not depend on your thirst to tell you to drink water. Try to drink at least 8 ounces of cool water for every 30 minutes of vigorous exercise.

CHAPTER 21

The Future of HIIT Workouts— 25 MORE Workouts!

I SINCERELY HOPE THAT YOU FIND ALL OF THESE WORKOUTS TO BE ENJOYABLE, CHALLENG- ing, and most importantly, health-enhancing. Hopefully, they will provide you with hours and hours of fitness bliss.

As to the future of HIIT training, I believe you will see many new HIIT programs and HIIT program variations in the coming months and years. HIIT training is definitely here to stay, and it will continue to evolve. In this chapter I'd like to introduce two new HIIT training programs that I think you will enjoy. The first is called "HIIT circuit training." This new workout style combines two popular exercise programs, HIIT training and circuit training. The other HIIT program is called "HIIT plus steady state." The development of these two new HIIT programs was founded on solid scientific research.

INTRODUCING HIIT CIRCUIT TRAINING

The HIIT circuit training program is an evolution of a safe way to combine HIIT workouts with muscle-strengthening workouts. Unfortunately, in the fitness industry some aggressive approaches of combining HIIT with muscular fitness exercises have resulted in harmful injures to participants. This will not happen with these HIIT circuit workouts. The combination of HIIT with circuit training is the grouping of two highly effective and time-efficient training programs. Circuit training is one of the most popular forms of muscle-strengthening training because you constantly move and change from one exercise to another exercise. No rest is needed between exercises because you are working different muscle groups. Also, you can complete the circuit 1, 2, 3, or more times. I have designed your circuit training exercises for the use of hand weights. Hand weights are inexpensive and easy to get from many commercial outlets. I suggest you start with lighter weights (such as 5-pound weights) and then progressively use heavier weights as you seek to challenge your muscles more. With each exercise, please complete the ascending (or lifting) motion in 2 seconds and the descending (or lowering) motion in 2 seconds. Breathe normally, not holding your breath, as you do the exercises.

HIIT CIRCUIT TRAINING EXERCISES

I'd like to introduce the circuit exercises, which will train all of your major muscle groups. For each exercise I tell you the area of the body that the exercise trains. The action instructs you how to do the exercise. The posture tip provides a key training tip related to body posture, and safe exercise movement. The variation suggestion provides a way you may choose to vary the exercise to change it up a little. To do a HIIT circuit training workout, please complete your HIIT workout first (whichever one from this book you are doing), and then complete your circuit workout. After you complete one exercise, move on to another. This circuit workout will only add about 10 more minutes to your training session. It is very time-efficient After you finish your circuit workout please go through your cooldown exercises. It is that easy! Let me teach you the correct form and technique for your circuit workout exercises.

SQUAT EXERCISE

This is a great exercise for the buttocks and thighs.

ACTION: Stand with feet placed slightly wider than your shoulders. Hold the hand weights next to your shoulders. Keeping your back straight, bend your legs and sit back with your buttocks as if you were sitting into a chair. Allow your buttocks to go the height of your knees and then return to the starting position. Complete 8–12 repetitions.

POSTURE TIP: As you sit back with your buttocks, try to keep your knees over your toes. This helps prevent any extra stress on the knee joint.

VARIATION SUGGESTION: With squats, regularly change the width of your stance to challenge your muscles with various standing positions.

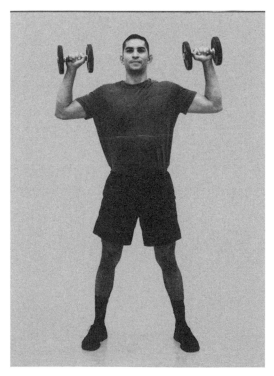
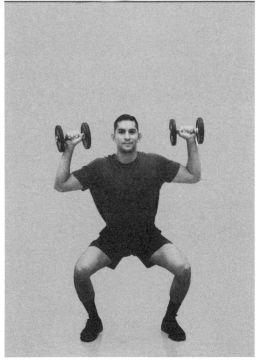

SHOULDER PRESS

This is a great exercise for the shoulders and back of the arms (triceps).

ACTION: Start in a standing position with your feet shoulder width apart. Place your hand weights next to your shoulders. Press the weights straight over your head and then return them to the starting position. Complete 8–12 repetitions.

POSTURE TIP: To keep your spine in alignment as you do the shoulder press, tighten your abdominal muscles, creating a muscular corset around the spine. This technique to protect the spine is called "bracing."

VARIATION: Alternate pressing one arm and then the other arm to concentrate on each arm.

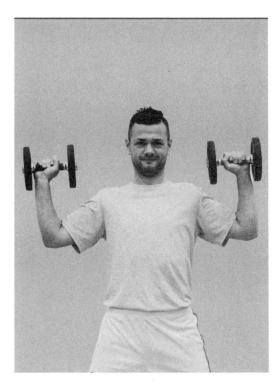
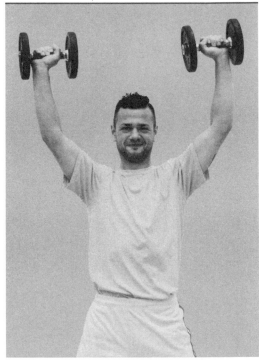

STEP FORWARD LUNGE

This is a great exercise for the thighs and buttocks.

ACTION: Stand with your feet together and hand weights down by your sides. Step forward about two to three feet with one leg bent at the knee. Keep the back leg extended, allowing it to bend slightly. Push back to a stand and repeat on the other leg. Complete 8–12 repetitions on each leg.

POSTURE TIP: As you perform the step forward lunge keep your back straight and the knee of the lunging leg over your toes.

VARIATION: For a greater muscular fitness challenge to the thighs and buttocks, do all of your repetitions on one side and then complete all of the repetitions on the other side.

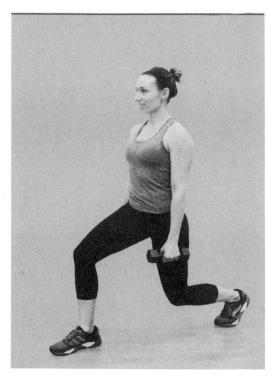 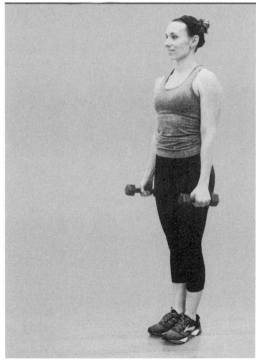

STANDING ROW

This is a great exercise for the upper and middle back.

ACTION: Stand with your legs shoulder width apart and your upper body slightly forward. Bend your knees slightly. Hold your hand weights to the sides of your legs. Pull your elbows as far back as they will go and then return to them to their starting position. Complete 8–12 repetitions.

POSTURE TIP: Do not bend forward too much, as this may overstress the spine.

VARIATION: Alternate pulling one arm as far back as you can, then return it to its starting position and complete with the other arm.

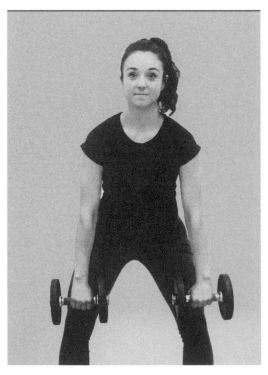 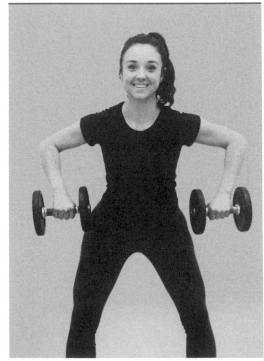

CHEST FLY

The is a great exercise for the chest and front part of the shoulders.

ACTION: Lie on a bench or floor with your hand weights extended directly over your shoulders. Keep a slight bend at your elbows. Slowly lower the arms perpendicularly away from your body and then back up to the starting position. Complete 8–12 repetitions.

POSTURE TIP: Keep your head steady and on the bench, so as not to stress your neck muscles during the exercise.

VARIATION: Alternate lowering and raising one arm at time to concentrate the effort in each arm.

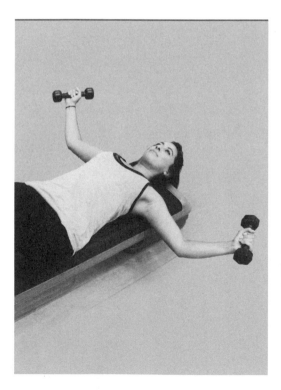 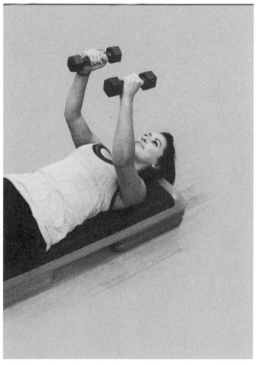

BICEP CURL

This is a great exercise for the front of the arms.

ACTION: Stand with legs shoulder width apart and knees slightly bent. Hold hand weights to the sides, arms extended, and palms facing away from the body. Bring the weights to the shoulders and then lower. Complete 8–12 repetitions.

POSTURE TIP: As you do the bicep curl motion keep your elbows next to the sides of your body.

VARIATION: Alternate lifting one arm and then the other arm.

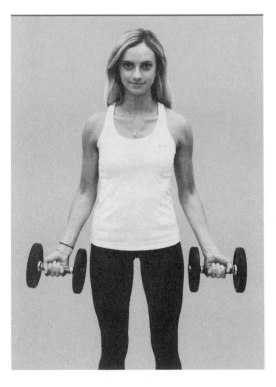
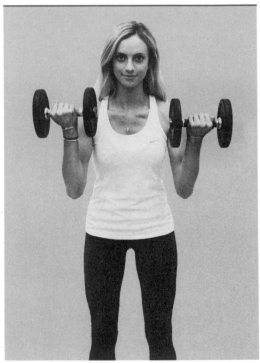

WIDE-ARM PUSH-UP

This is a great exercise for the back of the arms, chest, and core muscles of the spine. You will not need your hand weights for this exercise.

ACTION: Place your feet wider than shoulder width apart. Keep your fingers facing forward. Lower the body so your chest is within one inch of the floor. Extend back up to the starting position. Repeat 8–20 times.

POSTURE TIP: To really engage your core muscles, which protect your spine, tighten your abdominal muscles, creating a muscular corset around the spine (bracing).

VARIATION: Lift one leg off the ground while doing your push-ups to provide an even greater challenge. Regularly change the lifting leg.

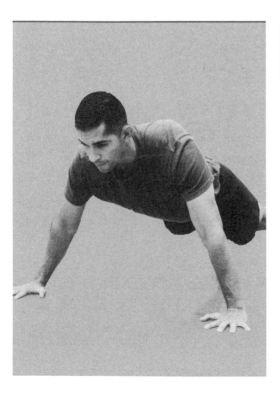 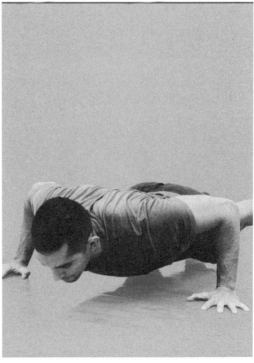

PLANK HOLD

The plank hold is a great exercise for the abdominals and core. You will not need your hand weights for this exercise.

ACTION: Start in a push-up position and then lower to both elbows on the ground. Hold this position for 30–45 seconds. Repeat the hold 3 times.

POSTURE TIP: Focus on keeping a straight line with your body from your ears to your knees. To keep the hips from sagging, give an extra squeeze to your buttocks. Make sure you breathe with slow, controlled breaths.

VARIATION: Gradually rock your weight over one arm and then back to the center, and then over the other arm. By changing the distribution of your weight from arm to arm, you challenge your core muscles more.

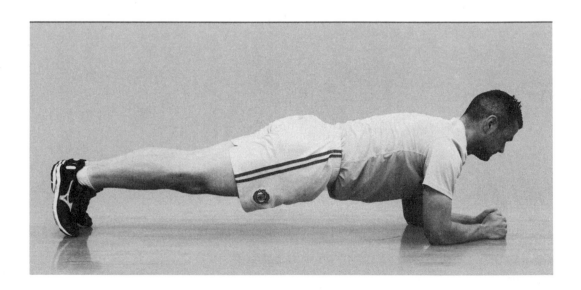

YOUR HIIT CIRCUIT WORKOUT PLAN

You can complete your HIIT circuit workouts whenever you wish to add a muscular fitness component to your workouts. In fact, on days you are not doing a HIIT workout, you can do your circuit workout by itself. I suggest you start with one circuit, completing the squat, shoulder press, step forward lunge, standing row, chest fly, bicep curl, wide-arm push-up, and plank hold. Go from one exercise to the other without any rest. Gradually progress and add a second, third, and even fourth circuit as you get stronger. When the weights feel too light for the number of repetitions, go ahead and get slightly heavier weighs. The American College of Sports Medicine (ACSM) recommends doing muscle-strengthening exercises of the major muscles of the body at least 2 times a week. That is a good goal. For variety in your circuit workout, I have designed five different circuit sequences, all using the same exercises. It is important to change up the exercise order to best continually stimulate your muscles. Here are the five circuits:

CIRCUIT 1: Perform exercises in this order: squat, shoulder press, step forward lunge, standing row, chest fly, bicep curl, wide-arm push-up, plank hold (complete 1–4 circuits).

CIRCUIT 2: Perform exercises in this order: shoulder press, step forward lunge, standing row, squat, chest fly, bicep curl, plank hold, wide-arm push-up (complete 1–4 circuits).

CIRCUIT 3: Perform exercises in this order: standing row, squat, shoulder press, step forward lunge, bicep curl, chest fly, wide-arm push-up, plank hold (complete 1–4 circuits).

CIRCUIT 4: Perform exercises in this order: step forward lunge, bicep curl, shoulder press, squat, standing row, chest fly, plank hold, wide-arm push-up (complete 1–4 circuits).

CIRCUIT 5: Perform exercises in this order: bicep curl, standing row, step forward lunge, shoulder press, squat, plank hold, chest fly, wide-arm push-up (complete 1–4 circuits).

> **SPECIAL REMINDER:** After you complete your circuit training please do your 5 stretches: calf and Achilles stretch, half-straddle stretch, quadriceps and hip flexors, lower back, abdominal, and chest stretch.

INTRODUCING HIIT PLUS STEADY-STATE WORKOUTS

I would like to share one more HIIT training program with you that will literally double the number of HIIT workouts presented in this book. In the scientific community, there's a lot of exciting discussion about combining HIIT workouts and steady-state workouts in a single training session. As you recall, steady-state exercise is comprised of continuous moderate-intensity aerobic workouts. There are countless health benefits to steady-state workouts, which are performed at a level 4 (somewhat hard) intensity on the perceived exertion intensity scale. As a result, many scientists believe that combining HIIT workouts with steady-state workouts is a promising new direction for cardiorespiratory health and function.

So, what's the plan for this combined HIIT–steady-state exercise? Here goes: after you complete any of the HIIT workouts presented in Chapter 20, you simply add a 10-minute steady-state workout to it immediately. You can do everything in the same mode (e.g., treadmill or cycle), or you can switch exercise modes during the steady-state segment. Here's an example where you switch: you do your HIIT workout on a treadmill and then complete the 10-minute steady-state workout on a cycle ergometer. That's it! You're limited only by whatever equipment is handy for you to use.

I call these new workouts "HIIT plus steady state", which is easy enough to remember. Plus, the HIIT plus steady state only adds an extra 10 minutes to your workout. That's really doable! Since the HIIT is the more challenging part of this workout, I recommend always completing the HIIT workout first, as you want to do your more demanding exercise earlier in your workout, when you are fresh. Here are two examples:

WORKOUT #21: 60S/90S HIIT PLUS STEADY STATE

TIMER SETTING: Set your timer to cue you ALTERNATELY at 60 seconds and 90 seconds.

EXERCISE MODE: Can be completed while walking, jogging, running, biking, elliptical striding, swimming, rowing, stair stepping, and/or using any type of cardio machine.

WARM-UP: Complete a 5–7 minute progressive warm-up at a perceived exertion intensity (PEI) level of 2–3 (light to mild-feeling intensity). Do the same exercise you will do for your HIIT workout.

HIIT WORKOUT DESIGN

	INTERVAL	DURATION	INTENSITY
BOUT 1	WORK Interval 1	60 seconds	PEI: Level 5: Feels challenging TALK Test: Moderate difficulty talking
	RECOVERY Interval 1	90 seconds	PEI: Level 2–4: Light movement to somewhat hard TALK Test: Mild to no difficulty talking
BOUT 2	WORK Interval 2	60 seconds	PEI: Level 5–6: Feels challenging to more challenging TALK Test: Moderate difficulty talking
	RECOVERY Interval 2	90 seconds	PEI: Level 2–4: Light movement to somewhat hard TALK Test: Mild to no difficulty talking

CHOOSE THE LENGTH OF THIS HIIT PLUS STEADY-STATE WORKOUT DEPENDING ON HOW YOU FEEL!

PROGRESSION: Please start off with the 10-minute HIIT workout.

- For a 10-minute workout complete 4 BOUTS
- Then, go right into the steady-state portion of the workout!

STEADY STATE: 10 minutes of steady state at a PEI level of 4 (somewhat hard intensity)

COOLDOWN: 3–5 minute progressive recovery at a mild intensity

DO YOUR 5 STRETCHES: Calf and Achilles Stretch, Half-Straddle Stretch, Quadriceps and Hip Flexors, Lower Back Stretch, Abdominal and Chest Stretch

WORKOUT #22: 60S/60S HIIT PLUS STEADY STATE

TIMER SETTING: Set your timer to cue you every 60 seconds.

EXERCISE MODE: Can be completed while walking, jogging, running, biking, elliptical striding, swimming, rowing, stair stepping, and/or using any type of cardio machine.

WARM-UP: Complete a 5–7 minute progressive warm-up at a perceived exertion intensity (PEI) level of 2–3, (light to mild-feeling intensity). Do the same exercise you will do for your HIIT workout.

HIIT WORKOUT DESIGN

	INTERVAL	DURATION	INTENSITY
BOUT 1	WORK Interval 1	60 seconds	PEI: Level 5: Feels challenging TALK Test: Moderate difficulty talking
	RECOVERY Interval 1	60 seconds	PEI: Level 2–4: Light movement to somewhat hard TALK Test: Mild to no difficulty talking
BOUT 2	WORK Interval 2	60 seconds	PEI: Level 5–6: Feels challenging to more challenging TALK Test: Moderate difficulty talking
	RECOVERY Interval 2	60 seconds	PEI: Level 2–4: Light movement to somewhat hard TALK Test: Mild to no difficulty talking

CHOOSE THE LENGTH OF THIS HIIT PLUS STEADY-STATE WORKOUT DEPENDING ON HOW YOU FEEL!

PROGRESSION: Please start off with the 10-minute HIIT workout.

- For a 10-minute workout complete 5 BOUTS
- Then, go right into the steady-state portion of the workout!

STEADY STATE: 10 minutes of steady state at a PEI level of 4 (somewhat hard intensity)

COOLDOWN: 3–5 minute progressive recovery at a mild intensity

DO YOUR 5 STRETCHES: Calf and Achilles Stretch, Half-Straddle Stretch, Quadriceps, and Hip Flexors, Lower Back Stretch, Abdominal and Chest Stretch

SUMMARY THOUGHTS

There you have it. You can do the HIIT plus steady-state workout with twenty HIIT workouts in this book, effectively giving yourself a total of forty workouts to choose from in *HIIT Your Limit*. I see a lot of sweat in your future. (And great health!) Speaking of the future, I believe it's only a matter of time until we will see some promising new research on these combined workouts. When you are ready to take your HIIT workouts to the next level, give these variations a try. The future is yours!

100 WINNING Ways to Cut Calories in Your Daily Life

IN MY MANY YEARS OF WORKING WITH EXERCISE ENTHUSIASTS AND PEOPLE TRYING TO LOSE weight, one of the most common questions I hear is, "What are some ways I can cut calories in my daily life?" Let's face it—regardless of the diet you're on or thinking of trying, cutting calories on a daily basis is a surefire way to lose weight. And, if you are doing your HIIT workouts regularly, you are going to lose mostly fat! That's because when you restrict calories in a safe way, exercise helps your body let go of more fat—precisely what you want. Cutting calories consistently but moderately is so much safer than the extreme weight loss approach advocated on *The Biggest Loser.* When it comes to weight management, losing weight gradually is the most successful strategy.

As you know from reading this book, my guiding philosophy for health, fitness, and weight management is, "Inch by inch, it's a cinch." I am confident that after making some of the easy, calorie-reducing changes in your daily life I suggest below, you will agree with this philosophy too. With this in mind, I proudly present to you: 100 winning ways to cut calories in your daily life. Before we get to them, a few notes:

1. Each tip has been validated by science, so rest easy.

2. To better help you navigate to specific questions you may have, I've organized this section into the following categories: Smart Swaps, Winning Behaviors to Follow in Your Daily Life, Winning Ideas to Follow at Home, and More Winning Ways to Cut Calories. Some of the winning ways cross over into a few categories, but I believe organizing them like this will maximize your reading enjoyment. I encourage you to highlight any ideas that jump out at you immediately—that way you can easily refer back to them. And then, of course, get to it!

SMART SWAPS

1. **MAKE SOME "SMART SWAPS" WHEN ORDERING MEALS AT A RESTAURANT.** When you go out to eat, do not hesitate to make special requests when you order. For instance, swapping vegetables for fries is a heart-healthy choice that really reduces the calories in your meal. Here are some other swaps: order grilled fish or chicken instead of fried. Perhaps try steamed or sautéed vegetables instead of potatoes in gravy. When ordering a burrito, smart

swap extra tomato and lettuce for the cheese. For a pasta smart swap, order pasta in olive oil instead of cream or meat sauce. Take control of your ordering by always being aware of healthy smart swaps you can make.

2. **USE LESS MAYONNAISE.** Adding mayonnaise to many foods, particularly sandwiches, is a common habit for a lot of people. Yet, most people are unaware of the consequences. In fact, only 1 tablespoon of mayonnaise will add >50 calories (depending on the brand) to your meal. If you enjoy using mayonnaise, try eating a bit less, or using light mayonnaise to reduce the number of calories you're eating.

3. **SPICE YOUR TEA OR COFFEE.** Tea and coffee are healthy, low-calorie drinks. I greatly enjoy my first cup of coffee each morning. How about you? However, adding just one teaspoon of sugar adds around 16 calories to your drink. I know; this doesn't sound like much. But, if you have 2 cups of coffee a day, that's at least 896 calories in one month. Wow—it adds up fast! Try using less sugar or perhaps substitute it with a small amount of a natural sugar-based sweetener like honey. Another option would be a natural, zero-calorie sweetener like stevia. Or even better, spice up your coffee and tea. Cinnamon helps stabilize blood sugar, and it's a good source of vitamin K and iron. You may wish to also try adding cardamom to your coffee. This warm, fragrant beverage is well liked in the Middle East, where cardamom seeds are often ground with coffee beans. Some people add whole cardamom pods or pre-ground cardamom powder to the brew. Start with one crushed *cardamom* pod per cup of *coffee*, and then fine-tune the quantity to your taste. Cardamom is a good source of vitamin C, calcium, magnesium, potassium, and zinc, and it also provides some dietary fiber, iron, and manganese.

4. **GO FOR THE MINIATURE VERSIONS OF SWEETS AND DESSERTS.** Lots of popular brands of ice creams, chocolates, and desserts now come in smaller mini sizes, as well as full-size versions. If you want a sweet treat, choose the smaller version of your favorite dessert and you will definitely avoid a lot of calories. Also, if you're eating out with a friend, family member, or companion, a great way to cut your portion size is by sharing your dessert. Plus, it's more enjoyable to share!

5. **ORDER APPETIZERS AS YOUR MEAL.** Overly large portions are a primary reason that people end up overeating in restaurants. If you're eating out and know that the restaurant serves large portions, you may be able to avoid overindulging by ordering a couple of healthy appetizers instead of a large meal. There's another benefit of this approach, too: it lets you enjoy a variety of tasty choices. Some healthy appetizer options may include steamed seafood (such as shrimp cocktail), salads that aren't loaded with cheese and bacon, grilled vegetables, and broth-based soups.

6. **DON'T UPGRADE.** Getting a larger drink or side dish for only a small increase in price may sound like a better deal. However, most restaurants already serve oversized food and drink portions, so stick to the regular size.

7. **SMART SWAP TOMATO-BASED SAUCES FOR CREAMY ONES.** A note to pasta lovers: creamy sauces not only contain more calories, they usually contain fewer vegetables as well. When preparing your pasta at home or choosing pasta at a restaurant, smart swap for a tomato-based sauce with vegetables over a creamy sauce and earn double benefits: fewer calories and more healthy vegetables.

8. **CHOOSE THE THIN CRUST.** Pizza is a popular fast food that can be very high in calories. If you want to enjoy some pizza, one way to keep the calories to a minimum is by choosing a thinner crust with lower-calorie toppings, such as vegetables.

9. **MOVE OVER MARGARITA.** I often frequent a favorite diner where I live, and when I'm there I notice many people savoring their happy hours with margaritas. More power to them, but many restaurants serve frozen margaritas in 18-ounce glasses—effectively tacking on over 400 calories to the meal that follows! Some restaurants now offer "skinny" margaritas, which have 50% fewer calories. If you enjoy margaritas with friends at a favorite bistro, see if the bartender will make you a skinny version.

10. **SIZE MATTERS WITH YOUR CAFFÈ LATTE.** A medium 18-ounce latte made with whole milk is 265 calories. A small 12-ounce latte made with fat-free milk is 125 calories. Making just this small modification in your choice of lattes will have a robust 130-calorie effect on your weight management success over the long run. Same great taste with a lot fewer calories.

11. **CHOOSE YOUR AFTERNOON DRINK WISELY.** A sweetened 16-ounce lemon iced tea from a vending machine has around 188 calories. Contrast this to sparkling water with natural lemon flavor (not sweetened), which has 0 calories. Both are very tasty. You can eliminate 188 calories each afternoon by opting for the sparkling water. Go for it.

12. **RETHINK YOUR DINNER BEVERAGE.** A glass of non-diet ginger ale (12 ounce) with your dinner meal adds 124 calories to your meal. Try smart swapping that with water with a slice of lemon or lime, which rings up at 0 calories. In 7 days that's an 868-calorie difference. These calories really add up! Rethinking your dinner beverage is a worthy objective for anyone with weight management goals.

13. **TRADE IN YOUR BACON AND EGG BREAKFAST ON AN ENGLISH MUFFIN.** Smart swap a grilled-veggie sandwich for that bacon and egg on an English muffin. A homemade bacon and egg on an English muffin with cheese has 22 grams of fat and 600 calories. Try replacing it with a grilled-vegetable (roasted peppers and spinach) toasted sandwich on whole grain bread. Not only does it taste delicious, but it's packed with nutrient-dense ingredients you're sure to enjoy.

14. **BUY PLAIN YOGURT.** Many people enjoy snacking on yogurt because of its protein content. The benefits of yogurt are impressive, but cartons full of fruit-flavored choices undo many of these bonuses (such as calcium) and add a lot of extra sugar calories. Feel free to top off your yogurt cup with a sprinkling of nuts and oats to complement the protein-rich treat.

15. **KNOW WHICH STEAKS HAVE THE MOST FAT.** You are definitely aware that fat adds flavor to food, particularly to steaks. But steaks have a wide range of fat content, and if you're watching your calories it is good to know the low-fat steaks versus the high-fat steaks. For

instance, 6-ounce servings of steaks that have >16 grams of fat include New York strip, porterhouse, T-bone, filet mignon, and rib eye. In contrast, 6-ounce portion size steaks with <12 grams of fat include top sirloin, bottom round, top round, and sirloin tip side steak. For the less tender steaks, lightly salt your meat at room temperature an hour before cooking it. The salt draws out the juices of the cut and tenderizes the protein, making it more flavorful and tender. Also, the extra-muscular fat on the outside of the steak—the gristle we typically do not eat—is easily trimmed off.

16. **EAT FRESH FRUIT.** Fresh fruit trumps fruit juice every time. Not only are fruit juices lacking in healthful fiber, they are also high in simple sugars. The edible skins of many fruits, including blueberries, apples, apricots, grapes, figs, plums, pears, prunes, raspberries, and strawberries have healthful carotenoids and flavonoids that fight off disease. Also, many fruit juices that are sold in supermarkets don't actually contain 100% fruit juice, and have added sweeteners such as sucrose and high fructose corn syrup. You should be aware of the calories in these fruit juices. For instance, a 12-ounce drink of 100% apple juice has 192 calories whereas an apple will have <70 calories (depending on its size). That is more than a 120-calorie difference—not to mention the many nutritional benefits of eating the whole fruit.

17. **HAVE A WHITE BUTTON MUSHROOM MEAL IN PLACE OF BEEF.** White button mushrooms are popularly consumed in the US and have been shown to improve heart health. They are available year-round and are served in various salads, soups, and casseroles, or eaten raw. A study in the journal *Appetite* found that eating a white bottom mushroom meal in place of a beef lunch reduced calorie intake by 420 calories. Wow! And, just as important, the study participants found the white button mushrooms lunch to be every bit as satisfying as the meat lunch.

18. **SMART SWAP A SPOONFUL OF SUGAR FOR CINNAMON.** When a recipe calls for sugar, you no longer have to think quickly for any substitutes, because you know spices are a great choice. Using spices like cinnamon or nutmeg, instead of excessive amounts of unnecessary sugar, is a great way to get tons of flavor without the extra calories, or the blood sugar spike. For example, instead of the two 50-calorie tablespoons of sugar you add to your plain morning oats, add a teaspoon of cinnamon at 6 calories. Plus it adds more taste!

19. **USE CAULIFLOWER INSTEAD OF RICE.** If you haven't already, it's time to start including cauliflower as one of the cruciferous (that is, member of the cabbage family) vegetables you eat on a regular basis. Some of the positive perks of cauliflower are that it is low-carb, low-calorie, and high in healthful phytonutrients! Remember, phytonutrients are the chemicals in plants that protect plants. Grating a cup of cauliflower to use in your rice recipe instead of using highly refined and nutrient-deficient white rice will save you 145 calories per cup.

20. **USE A GOURMET OIL SPRAYER.** One of the keys to using any oil with a meal is to use it in moderation, especially since a tablespoon of oil has around 125 calories. Gourmet oil sprayers are designed with the health-conscious person in mind. These sprayers make it easy to mist your favorite oil on an entire dish without overdoing it. It offers a way to add flavor and use less oil, and it easily saves you over 50 calories compared to pouring straight out of the bottle.

21. **STIR-FRY WITH CHICKEN BROTH.** Soy sauce has around 900 milligrams of sodium per tablespoon, and low-sodium soy sauce has more than 500 milligrams of sodium in 1 tablespoon. Despite this, you don't have to eliminate stir-fry cooking from your diet. Try adding a couple of tablespoons of low-sodium chicken broth to your skillet instead and get it nice and hot. Add veggies and stir—it's that easy. You'll save a lot of calories and use much less salt in the process!

22. **POACH YOUR EGGS.** Poaching your eggs is a fat-free cooking method that saves at least 50 calories compared to using half a tablespoon of butter to cook them another way. Poached eggs are lower in calories and fat than eggs that have been fried, scrambled, or baked, all of which require oil or butter.

23. **SMART SWAP APPLES FOR CRACKERS.** For your next wine and cheese get together, pair your cheddar cheese cubes with slices of apples sprinkled with a little lemon (to keep them from going brown), instead of crackers. This healthy swap replaces refined carbohydrates in

crackers with slow-digesting healthy complex carbs (in the apple slices). Plus, you get extra vitamins, fiber, and a sweet complement to your cheese, besides saving a lot of calories.

24. **JUST EAT HALF OF YOUR BURRITO.** Let's face it: many of us enjoy the countless tasty offerings at the fast casual Mexican grills that proliferate across the country. I grew up in New Mexico and am quite fond of Mexican cuisine. Yet, a typical meat burrito with cheese, salsa, lettuce, sour cream, rice, and beans may have more than 1,000 calories, plus almost a full day's worth of sodium, and a lot of saturated fat. *Wow*—that is just too much tastiness if you are trying to manage your weight. One option to significantly lower the calories is to eat half the order in a bowl and then take the rest home for another meal. Did you know that not eating the large tortilla will also drop up to 400 calories, depending on the size and type of tortilla?

25. **SQUASH YOUR SPAGHETTI.** Instead of pouring a box of highly refined spaghetti into a pot of boiling water, try baking a spaghetti squash. You'll up the number of veggies you eat *and* slash calories in the process. The string-like squash has only 31 calories per cup, as compared to 318 calories in a cup of penne pasta. That's almost 300 calories you can save!

26. **HAVE VEGGIES WITH YOUR BURGER.** Whether you're having your favorite beef burger, portabella mushroom burger, or veggie burger, have healthy veggies for your side dish. Instead of fries or chips, which may have over 400 calories in a serving, try roasted potatoes, roasted sweet potatoes, Mexican corn salad, coleslaw, mango black bean salad, cucumber salad, red cabbage salad, or some of your other favorite vegetables.

27. **USE SPICES INSTEAD OF SAUCES.** We all look for ways to add some extra flavor to an otherwise bland meal. Instead of adding extra sauce, why not use spices instead? Spices add flavor, but they do it without adding major calories and unhealthy sugars to your meal. For instance, the herb oregano goes wonderfully well with pizza and pasta. It is a widespread ingredient in many Greek recipes as well. Oregano has a zesty bite and slight peppery edge that will make any dish a little more savory.

28. **DO YOU KNOW ABOUT THE "SALAD ADD-ON DANGER ZONE"? DRIED FRUIT, BACON BITS, CHEESE, AND CROUTONS ADD A LOT OF FLAVOR TO A SALAD, BUT THEY ALSO ADD CALORIES.** If you are thinking about adding them, you are in what's benevolently called the "salad add-on danger zone." For example, dried fruit becomes quite calorie-dense in the dehydrating process. It also has added sugar and oil. Go with fresh blueberries, grapes, and apples instead. Bacon bits are processed meat, which is associated with colorectal cancer. Smart swap out the bacon bits with beans or chickpeas, which add flavor and protein. Go light on the cheese, as it is a big source of saturated (unhealthy) fat in the diet that promotes cardiovascular disease and type 2 diabetes. Perhaps look for a nut-based cheese as a smart swap. Croutons add that enjoyable crunch to a salad, and some calories, but have no nutritional benefit. A piece of whole grain bread is a much better smart swap. Toast it and sprinkle it on the salad for that crunchy taste.

29. **TRY SOME ANCIENT GRAINS.** When you read about eating more whole grains, you typically think of whole wheat bread, barley, brown rice, and oatmeal. However, there are some other healthy options known as ancient grains nudging their way onto mainstream supermarket shelves. Ancient grains have not been changed by selective breeding over the years, as have been most cereals, corn, rice, and varieties of wheat. These ancient grains include amaranth, *Kamut, freekeh,* farro, teff, and quinoa, and are well worth a try. Plus, they are filled with B vitamins, magnesium, potassium, iron, fiber, and protein. Give them a go and see which ones you like.

30. **YOU DON'T HAVE TO SKIP DESSERT WHEN YOU GO OUT.** Dining out is a culinary pleasure for all of us to enjoy. However, people on restricted diets feel they always have to eliminate the dessert. This needn't be. You can be savvy with your dessert choices. Restaurant brownies, slices of cake, and other baked items often contain more fat and calories than you might consume in an entire day. Instead, smart swap angel food cake for the traditional desserts. Request that your server top it with fresh fruit. The fruit will provide potassium, vitamin C, and fiber. Also, many eateries now have mini baked desserts, which are often served in a small shot glass. They are considerably lower in calories than their full-size counterparts.

Low-fat frozen yogurt is an agreeable smart swap for ice cream, particularly with some fresh fruit. When at home, go for some chopped fresh fruit, low-fat yogurt and a light sprinkle of nuts. That's a real sweet treat.

31. **HERE'S A TACO MEAL MAKEOVER THAT WORKS.** There is no reason to skip the tacos—just tweak your menu. Wrap your taco filling in corn tortillas rather than flour ones, then top off each with a tablespoon of sour cream, plus salsa with half a slice of cheddar cheese. Corn tortillas, at 62 calories per tortilla, are typically much smaller than large flour tortillas, which pack a whopping 467 calories per tortilla. This taco meal makeover will spare you over 300 calories.

32. **SERVE SOME HEALTHY PARTY FOODS.** When hosting a party, steer away from giving your guests those mozzarella sticks with dipping sauce. Instead, go with bruschetta. It's one of the healthier party foods to make. Just add a mixture of tomatoes, olive oil, garlic, and basil to thinly sliced, toasted Italian bread and presto—you've got bruschetta. The tomatoes contain lycopene, a potent antioxidant found to ward off heart disease and cancer.

33. **HAVE A LITTLE POPCORN ON FAMILY MOVIE NIGHT.** On home theater night with family and friends, a little popcorn is mighty fine. The popcorn hull, the part that gets stuck in your teeth, is a nutritional powerhouse. It contains polyphenols, which are healthy antioxidants. Those antioxidants help to deactivate those harmful cellular free radical molecules. Pass on the microwaveable stuff and instead go with air-popped popcorn, which is high in fiber, low in calories, and contains no sugar or sodium.

34. **HAVE A BOTTLED YOGURT SMOOTHIE FOR A SNACK.** If you are on the go and need a quick snack, have a bottled yogurt smoothie. But first, check the label. If it lists fructose or high fructose corn syrup as one of the first ingredients, don't choose it. It has too much sugar.

35. **BALANCE YOUR MEALS WITH FRUITS AND VEGGIES.** If most of your meals consist of meat and potatoes or pasta and cheese, you should try to balance these high-calorie choices

with more fresh produce. You'll learn to relish fruits and veggies in no time. Try this idea: balance your breakfast by making it half fruit, and do the same with your lunch and dinner by making it half veggie. That's an achievable healthy balance.

36. **A CHOCOLATE SNACK YOU MAY ENJOY.** I have always been a fan of chocolate. In my travels around the world I have tasted many wonderful and exotic chocolates. However, for a feel-good, comfort food snack at home, I go with chocolate-covered pretzels. They are not that nutrient-dense, but I like to consider them as a backup snack when I desire a little chocolate.

37. **LOVE YOUR CHILI.** A serving, one cup, of a typical canned chili has 287 calories. A cup of turkey chili is 224 calories and a cup of veggie chili is right around 200 calories. By not adding a slice of cheddar cheese you will be saving 113 calories. However, please avoid the salsa chips. A cup of them is 293 calories and 539 milligrams of sodium. Have you tried cucumber slices as a smart swap for the chips? They're really tasty and there are only 8 calories in a bowl of cucumber slices.

WINNING BEHAVIORS TO FOLLOW IN YOUR DAILY LIFE

38. **DON'T DRINK YOUR CALORIES.** Drinks can be a forgotten source of calories in your diet. Sugar-sweetened drinks such as soda are high in calories. They're also linked to obesity and the development of type 2 diabetes. A single 16-ounce bottle of cola can contain nearly 200 calories, including about 44 grams of sugar. One study indicates that drinking lots of sugar-sweetened beverages not only adds heaps of unnecessary calories to your diet, it may also increase your hunger later on in the day.

39. **CHOOSE A LOW-CALORIE MEAL STARTER.** Research shows that choosing a low-calorie meal starter such as salad or soup may help prevent overeating. In fact, one study found that enjoying soup before a main meal could lessen the total amount of calories you eat during the meal by as much as 20%. Let's do the numbers. If you ordered a 600-calorie meal, you could potentially cut 120 calories just by having the salad. Remember, with weight management, it's all about finding ways that work for you. This seems really doable.

40. **ORDER SALAD DRESSINGS ON THE SIDE.** Often what begin as healthy, low-calorie salads become deceptively high in calories due to the amount of salad dressing in them. Enjoy your salad dressing, but order it on the side so you can control the amount used.

41. **BE WARY OF ALL-YOU-CAN-EAT BUFFETS AND SALAD BARS.** It goes without saying that portion sizes often get way out of control in restaurants offering to give customers more food for their dollar. We consumers have been programmed into thinking that bigger size means better value. Challenged with sizeable amounts of food at a meal, most people are more likely to overeat. Indeed, this is an obstacle you face at all-you-can-eat buffets and salad bars, where it is easy to overindulge. Try to reduce the number of returns back to the buffet bar. If you know dining at an all-you-can-eat buffet leads to overeating for you, try to avoid going to them.

42. **GOODBYE BREADBASKET.** When you're hungry, it's easy to reach for the pre-dinner bread at a restaurant and start nibbling. Serving bread is a friendly way to welcome a customer, while also giving patrons something to snack on prior to the arrival of their ordered food. This habit of eating bread and the butter before a meal can add hundreds of calories. In fact, one slice of white bread with butter is 116 calories. And, the bread may actually make you hungrier. Yes, the carbohydrates in bread may trigger insulin production, which makes you even hungrier. Send the breadbasket back or request that your server not even bring bread to the table. Similarly, when eating at a Mexican restaurant, use moderation when enjoying the pre-dinner chips.

43. **PRUNE YOUR MEAL.** One way to cut a few calories is to literally trim the meal you have chosen to eat. For example, if you're eating a burger, taking off the bun will save you around 160 calories, and perhaps even more if the bun is really big. You can even shave a few calories off your sandwich by removing one slice of bread to make yourself a special open sandwich. This idea of pruning your meals is remarkably easy to do!

44. **BE MINDFUL OF YOUR ALCOHOL DRINKING.** There's nothing wrong with appreciating a drink or two. But my suggestion is to just be mindful of the calories in the alcohol you

consume, as well as the amount you're consuming. There are plenty of apps that give you caloric values of your favorite drinks. For instance, one vodka soda is about 65 calories versus one rum and coke, which is about 250 calories. That's about a 200-calorie difference, which is a lot!

45. **EAT MORE WHOLE FRUITS.** Whole fruits contain lots of fiber, vitamins, minerals, and antioxidants. Accordingly, whole fruits should be a prominent, healthy portion of your diet. And, compared with fruit juice, whole fruits are difficult to over consume, because they fill you up. Whenever possible, choose whole fruits over fruit juice. They're more filling and contain more nutrients with fewer calories.

46. **TAKE OFF THE SKIN ON YOUR CHICKEN SELECTIONS.** Eating the skin on your chicken adds extra calories to your meal. For example, a skinless roasted chicken breast is around 142 calories. The same chicken breast with skin contains 193 calories, or about 50 extra calories. Go skinless chicken for fewer calories.

47. **WEAN YOURSELF FROM SECONDS.** Often a meal is so delicious that you are tempted to have seconds of a serving. This may be one of the bigger challenges you may face with your eating behaviors. I know this is a challenge I regularly battle. First, be aware that a second serving often leads to eating more calories than you need. Chances are the first helping was satisfactory. Although you can feel your stomach filling up as you eat, it can take up to 20 minutes after food is eaten before the satiety signals reach your brain. Try eating a little slower and see if this helps to wean you off a second serving. Also, alcohol may stimulate appetite in the short-term with some people, and therefore encourage more eating. Set a priority goal to wean yourself from seconds. You can do it, but take it one meal at a time. Remember, "Inch by inch, it's a cinch."

48. **YOUR EMOTIONS AFFECT YOUR EATING.** There are several books and plenty of articles on emotional eating. Have you done any reading on the topic? If you haven't, it's quite intriguing. Here are some points to remember: research shows that people experience

higher levels of hunger during moments of anger and joy, as opposed to moments of fear and sadness. In addition, people tend to become impulsive eaters during moments of anger. Also, people tend to make healthier food choices when they are feeling joyful. Yes, your emotions definitely affect your eating behaviors.

49. **EAT MORE FIBER.** Many weight loss experts encourage patients to eat more fiber for successful weight loss. Fiber is a carbohydrate found in plant foods like whole grains, vegetables, and fruits. Unlike other carbs, your body doesn't readily digest fiber, so it passes through your system without triggering your blood sugar to rise. There's nothing magical about foods with fiber; they just keep you full longer without adding extra calories to your diet. Women should get about 25 grams a day and men at least 35 to 40. The average American, however, gets just 15 grams a day of fiber. Some options to consider are whole grain breads, brown rice, black beans, low-fat popcorn, oranges, raisin bran cereal, oatmeal and fresh strawberries.

50. **USE SOME COMMON REFERENCE POINTS TO HELP GAUGE HEALTHY PORTION SIZES.** When it comes down to it, most people are just unsure about what normal portion sizes look like. This is because fast food, casual cuisine, and high-end eateries serve rather large portions. Let's go over a few tips you can remember: a clenched fist or baseball is equivalent to about one cup. A large egg or light bulb would be about half a cup. The tip of your thumb would be one teaspoon. A poker chip would be about one tablespoon. A golf ball is about one ounce. You can go to choosemyplate.gov for more information on various portion sizes and other nutrition resources.

51. **DAB YOUR PIZZA.** Yes, dab your pizza to make your slice a little more waistline-friendly. All you have to do is press down on the pizza slice with a paper napkin to absorb the orangey grease. That grease is excess fat from the fatty cheese that rises to the top after being cooked. A study by *Labdoor Magazine* found that dabbing the oil from the surface of your slice with a paper towel or napkin can wipe away 40 calories and 4.5 grams of fat per slice (compared to an un-dabbed one). Have two slices and you've saved 80 calories! The *Labdoor* study

report estimates that the average American eats 23 pounds of pizza per year. Therefore, dabbing the oil off each slice you eat can lead to an estimated 2 pounds of fat weight loss per year. It's not a large number, but it exemplifies the small changes approach, which I call "Inch by inch, it's a cinch." In the long run, it's all of the small changes you make—and sustain—that lead to weight loss success and weight regain prevention.

52. **SPLITTING MEALS SAVES CALORIES AND MONEY.** An easy way to meaningfully reduce calories, and enjoy your meal, is to share your entree at the restaurant with a friend, family member, or companion. Most restaurant meal portion sizes are quite large, and by splitting the meal you may be able to really enjoy the offering, save some money, and not have to pay the consequence of too many calories.

53. **STAY AWAY FROM PROBIOTICS THAT CLAIM WEIGHT LOSS BENEFITS.** Probiotics are bacteria that we eat for health. They are microorganisms that, when taken in adequate amounts, have some medicinal benefits, such as improving immune function, protecting against hostile bacteria to prevent infection, and improving digestion and absorption of food and nutrients. If the balance between bad and good gut bacteria is disturbed, worrisome health problems may occur. This imbalance is often caused by taking a lot of antibiotics; so, if an imbalance happens, probiotics may help restore some of the good bacteria in the gut. The current use of probiotics for weight loss, however, is an area full of debate and controversy. Although there are numerous probiotic products that claim weight loss benefits, the research doesn't fully support these claims at this time. Save your pennies and hold off on purchasing probiotics that claim weight loss benefits.

54. **MAKE A PLAN TO EAT.** With weight management, it is very helpful to plan when you are going to eat. Know what you plan to eat and then stick to the plan. Yes, this may sound like a novel idea, but it works; having no plan is the equivalent of planning to fail. In addition, I always encourage the students I teach to schedule their workouts and guard that time as if it were non-negotiable. It shows you have a lot of self-respect for your quality of life.

55. **GET FANCY WITH SOME HEALTHY SAUCES AND DRESSING.** You have plenty of great options when it comes to low calorie sauces and salad dressings. For instance, smart swap tomato sauce instead of Alfredo on pasta, or smart swap hummus or mustard for mayo on a sandwich. With salad dressings, be a little adventuresome. Trying sprinkling your favorite fruits and nuts as a salad dressing. Or how about some fresh apricots and apple cider vinegar mixed with a little Dijon mustard for another savory dressing? Be creative and go for it.

56. **HAVE SOME PEANUT BUTTER.** Peanut butter is a great source of protein, healthy fats, and fiber. Please note, a low-calorie serving size is two level tablespoons, which is 188 calories. Perhaps add a tablespoon of peanut butter to a fruit smoothie and enjoy.

57. **MID-AFTERNOON SNACKS ARE BETTER THAN MID-MORNING SNACKS.** If you are going to have a snack, choose the mid-afternoon. There is less time between breakfast and lunch than there is between lunch and dinner. In some cases, mid-morning snacks can become mindless habits. If you do have a mid-morning snack, make it a snack-walk. Get your 3 minutes (or more) of movement, before or after the snack.

WINNING IDEAS TO FOLLOW AT HOME

58. **COOK YOUR OWN FOOD WHEN POSSIBLE.** When you buy food prepared at an eatery, you don't always know what's in it. Sometimes meals that you think are healthy or low-calorie can contain hidden sugars and fats, bumping up their calorie content. Cooking your own food will give you better control over what's going into your meals. People who cook dinner at home consume about 140 fewer calories than when they dine out or order in. When possible, stay home and cook.

59. **DON'T KEEP JUNK FOOD IN THE HOUSE.** If you buy unhealthy food by habit, or if there is a special offer on it, you typically end up eating it. It is best not to have it in your house. Think about it. There are times when you are in a big rush or you are voraciously hungry. This is the time you need to choose from the healthy options and not be tempted to eat the available junk food. Make your environment a healthier one for you. You are worth it.

60. **USE SMALLER PLATES.** Today's dinner plates are, on average, approximately 44% larger than they were in the 1980s. Interestingly, larger plates have been linked with larger serving sizes, which means you are more likely to overeat. In fact, one study found that at a buffet, people with larger dinner plates ate 45% more food than those who used the smaller plate size. Choosing a smaller plate is a simple tactic that can keep your portion sizes on track and help you curb overeating.

61. **INCREASE THE VEGETABLE PORTION OF YOUR MEALS.** Most people don't eat enough vegetables. In fact, it's estimated that around 87% of people in the US don't eat the recommended amount. That's a staggering statistic! Letting vegetables fill up a large portion of your plate is a first-rate way to cut back on higher-calorie foods. Choose vegetables such as kale, spinach, carrots, broccoli, peas, asparagus, brussels sprouts, scallions, zucchini, green beans, cauliflower, green bell peppers, okra, avocado, and corn.

62. **EAT YOUR MEALS SLOWLY AND TAKE SMALLER BITES.** With every meal, take your time to chew your foods slowly. For many people this easy technique has been shown to help them eat less at a meal. Also, try taking smaller bites. It may also help you eat less in the long run.

63. **EAT WITHOUT DISTRACTIONS AT HOME.** This is quite fascinating: studies show your dining environment plays a profound role in how much you eat on a daily basis. The research indicates that if you're distracted while you eat, you're prone to overeat. Isn't that interesting? One recent research review found that people who were distracted while eating consumed 30% more food compared to others who were mindful about their meal. Unhealthy distractions to avoid while you're eating include watching TV, using your cell phone, playing computer games, reading a book, or working at your computer. How many of these do you do while eating? Want to make a change? Go for it!

64. **TRY MINDFUL EATING.** We in the US have been conditioned to eat everything placed in front of us. Many people put food into their mouths almost unconsciously. Instead, try mindful eating. This means eating with attention to improve your eating behaviors. Mindful eating is the practice of cultivating an open-minded awareness of how the food you choose to eat affects your feelings and thoughts. With successful mindful eating awareness, you will likely make healthy food choices in your meals and eat until you're satisfied, and not just full.

65. **INCLUDE PROTEIN WITH MORE OF YOUR MEALS.** Eating a little more protein in your meals is considered a useful strategy for weight loss and weight regain prevention. As discussed earlier in this book, foods higher in protein use more energy to digest and can fill you up more than other nutrients, like fat and carbohydrates. Of course, make sure the rest of your meal has a good mix of fresh fruits, vegetables, and whole grains. There is recent research that increased protein with a meal will lead to greater satiety, weight loss, fat mass loss, and the preservation of muscle. Some suggestions for protein-rich foods include fish, poultry, beans, legumes, nuts, tofu, eggs, and low-fat or non-fat dairy products.

66. **SKIP THE EXTRA CHEESE.** When preparing your meals, you might add extra cheese to a sandwich or dish. I know I regularly deal with this challenge. Skip it. Even a single slice of cheese can add around 100 calories to your meal.

67. **MODIFY YOUR COOKING METHODS.** Cooking your own meals is a great way to keep your meals healthy and your calorie intake under control. However, if you're trying to cut back on calories, then some cooking methods are better than others. For instance, a good way to cut down on the number of extra calories you're adding to your food is by boiling, grilling, poaching, or steam frying as opposed to traditional frying in oils.

68. **SUPER-PROCESSED FOODS ARE OUT.** Super-processed foods like lunch meats, chips, pancake syrup, candy bars, cookies, cakes, fruit juices, and sweetened coffees have lots of calories and often make you hungrier. Take an inventory of how many of these foods are part of your daily life and start minimizing that list.

69. **DIP VEGETABLES, NOT CHIPS.** It's OK to snack, but eating chips and dips while watching TV is not your best option. For instance, carrots with hummus are a healthy and delicious snack. Cucumbers with hummus are also quite tasty. Be mindful that pretzels are lower in calories and fat than chips and also have trace amounts of certain vitamins and minerals. But pretzels are high in sodium, so be mindful of how many you eat! Additionally, for you chip fans, there are some new, healthy bean chip and lentil chip options on the market that appear to be growing in popularity.

70. **EAT YOUR BEEF WITH GREENS.** Do you enjoy eating beef? Then enjoy your favorite steak, chili, or stew. However, try serving it over a bed of greens, like baby kale, spinach, or beet greens in place of mashed potatoes, pasta, or rice.

71. **HAVE YOUR SANDWICH ON A SALAD.** For those of you who enjoy variety in your meals try this: put your sandwich, without the bread and mayo, on a salad. Two big slices of bread with mayo can tally up to 550 calories. That is a lot of calories. Try this sandwich on a salad option—it really tastes delicious.

72. **STAY AWAY FROM THE DARK SIDE—EATING LATE AT NIGHT.** Do you enjoy late-night munchies? Let's face it: many people tell me they hear the refrigerator calling their name late at night. I think I have heard those calls too—usually around midnight! Yes, I do know what it is like to be a midnight muncher. Scientists tell us it is not so much the timing that matters, but the choice of foods people select late at night. For instance, favorite after-dark, late-evening choices include chocolate, ice cream, potato chips, and desserts. All choices with too many calories! Please laser focus for a moment. This habit has got to go if you are going to lose weight and permanently keep it off. Take this message to heart and remember: late-night munching packs on the pounds. Time to say goodbye!

73. **CUT BACK ON PAN-FRYING OIL.** Pan-frying at home is a routine cooking technique that uses a large amount of oil. A tablespoon of oil is 120 calories. Best advice: no matter which oil you choose, use as little as possible. One heart-healthy oil option is extra virgin olive oil. Extra virgin olive oil (the highest quality olive oil with the best flavor) also contains beta-carotene and vitamins A, E, D, and K, and many more healthful nutrients. Studies show these nutrients have favorable effects on almost every bodily function.

74. **BREAKFAST IS A WINNER MEAL.** Have a modest breakfast each morning. Doing so is a very common practice among the ten thousand plus men and women in the National Weight Control Registry, all of whom have lost at least 30 pounds and kept it off for over one year. Also, research shows that people who skip breakfast are more prone to obesity. Plan for a healthy breakfast each and every morning. What's for breakfast tomorrow? Always good to plan ahead!

75. **EAT BREAKFAST WITHIN 2 HOURS OF AWAKENING.** Eating within 2 hours of awakening will make a difference in the way you process blood sugar all day. Research is finding that maintaining glucose and insulin in the right balance has important effects on metabolism, body weight and health.

76. **INVEST IN NONSTICK COOKWARE.** Using nonstick cookware allows food to be browned without sticking to the pan. Plus, it will save on calories. For instance, when you fry an

egg in a nonstick pan, as compared to a traditional cast-iron skillet, you'll save at least 50 calories from not having to use cooking oil.

77. **START BAKING WITH APPLESAUCE.** Whether it's in cakes, brownies, or cookies—when you're baking, just substitute unsweetened applesauce for oil in a 1:1 ratio in your recipe. For instance, 1/4 cup of canola oil is almost 500 calories, where as a 1/4 cup of unsweetened applesauce is 26 calories. That is a 475-calorie difference. Simply replace the melted oil with an equal amount of applesauce. You may need to bake things longer when using applesauce, but it will be well worth it.

78. **HAVE A "NICE CREAM" DESSERT.** Nice cream is a creamy dessert that resembles ice cream but is made entirely with frozen bananas and any added toppings you select. It is the perfect way to satisfy your sweet tooth while laser focusing on your weight management goals. To make it, add two frozen bananas to a blender with a tablespoon of unsweetened cocoa powder and blend until you reach that creamy consistency of soft-serve ice cream. Spoon into a bowl and enjoy. Or, freeze for about 15 more minutes for a taste that rivals your favorite ice cream. You are going to like this guiltless calorie treat. Share it with your friends!

79. **DON'T EAT FROM THE BAG.** It's much harder to keep track of your calories when you eat right from the bag. Yes, you know what I mean—it could be a bag of chips, crackers, or cookies. When you eat from the bag, you tend to continue eating until your food is gone. (And if you're eating from a large bag that could be a lot of food.) Be more focused on your portion control. If you decide to have some chips, cookies, or crackers, take out the amount you feel is a healthy portion size and place it on a plate. Then, put the bag back in the cupboard. Full disclosure: I am a recovering cookie bag aficionado. This approach works for me and I am sure it will work for you too!

80. **EAT MORE FATTY FISH.** Fatty fish, like salmon, mackerel, herring, lake trout, sardines, and albacore tuna, have generous portions of omega-3 fatty acids. Omega-3 fatty acids are healthy and may help reduce your circulating cortisol levels in the blood. This is great,

because elevated levels of cortisol are closely associated with depositing fat in your middle area. Please, no more belly fat.

MORE WINNING WAYS TO CUT CALORIES

81. **TRY THE 80% EATING STYLE.** One of the healthiest populations on the planet are men and women from Okinawa, Japan. They often live to be 100 years and beyond. They follow a practice called *hara hachi bu*, which means "eat until you are 80% full." Of course, it helps to eat healthy food as well! One challenge: what does it feels like to be 80% full? Start by eating half of what you normally eat, and then assess how you feel. When you start to feel a little stomach pressure you're right about at 80% full. You will eventually discover the difference between eating to a point of no longer feeling hungry (80% full) and eating to a point of fullness.

82. **MONITOR YOUR FOOD INTAKE WITH A TECHNOLOGY PAL.** Even if only for a few days, keep track of what you eat in a journal or app. When you do this, keep track of the calorie count for each meal. Many people discover patterns of eating that they can change once they become aware of their typical eating behaviors. There are several apps that you can use, like Lose It!, MyFitnessPal, and MyPlate.

83. **ASK YOUR WAITER TO BOX UP HALF OF YOUR MEAL BEFORE IT GETS TO THE TABLE.** Recent research indicates that excess energy intake from meals consumed away from home is a major contributor to the obesity epidemic. According to a new study, boxing up half your meal before it arrives can save up to 600 calories for one outing.

84. **ROTATE YOUR MEALS.** Since foods contain so many different nutrients it's a good idea to establish some type of meal rotation so that you consume a wide range of nutritional benefits. For instance, there are many cereals that are high in fiber and low in sugar. Add some fruit to them to complete the meal, but be sure to regularly rotate your fruit choices. For lunch, rotating meals more frequently is easy. Need ideas? How about rotating salads with low-calorie dressings, sandwiches on whole grain bread (minus the mayo), and broth-based

soups. Again, rotate some of your favorite sides of vegetable. For dinner, rotate some healthy meals that include foods like chicken, fish, and whole grains. You can get pretty creative with your meal rotations.

85. **DRINK WATER BEFORE YOUR MEAL.** Drinking water before a meal may help you feel more satisfied, prompting you to eat fewer calories. For example, one 2015 study in the journal *Obesity* showed that drinking two 8-ounce cups of water 20–30 minutes prior to a meal lowered calorie intake by about 13%. Why not see if drinking water before your meals helps you attain and maintain your weight management goals? It is worth a try.

86. **PUT YOUR PHONE AWAY DURING LUNCH.** A 2011 study published in the *American Journal of Clinical Nutrition* found that playing a computer game during lunch led to eating more at lunch and more at a subsequent meal. Because of the distraction, people were less aware of how much food they were consuming. For better or worse—probably for worse—we live in a multitasking society, and many of us often eat our meals while watching TV or using our mobile devices. Try paying attention to what you're eating and turn off those devices: you are more likely to eat less during that meal and the next one, too.

87. **START FIDGETING MORE AS YOU SIT.** Yes, that's correct. This isn't a way to cut calories, but an easy way to burn more calories. For many years, I have been encouraging students to fidget whenever they can during the day, particularly when they are sitting. When you fidget while seated, you burn up to 54% more calories than when you are seated motionless. That is a BIG difference! You probably are thinking, what are the best ways to fidget? Try these options. When sitting, periodically alternate extending your legs off the floor. Next, while sitting normally, alternate rotating your torso to the right and left. In addition, periodically raise your arms over your head, one at a time, and allow your torso to turn as you lift an arm. Find a nice rhythm to regularly incorporate these movements into your sustained sitting times. My students often ask me how many times they should do a movement. I always say, start with three and add more when you want. And don't forget, for every 30 minutes of sitting, get your 3 minutes (or more) of movement.

88. **ARRIVE LATE TO HAPPY HOUR AND LEAVE EARLY.** It's too easy to pack on pounds at happy hour. Alcohol has more calories (7 calories per gram) compared to carbohydrates and protein, which have 4 calories per gram. And when you drink moderately at happy hour you are also less likely to eat some of that high calorie bar food. Stick to one or two drinks at happy hour by arriving late and leaving early.

89. **DON'T SHOP WHEN YOU'RE HUNGRY.** This suggestion is really helpful. You'll be less likely to put tempting foods into your shopping cart if you shop when you're *not* hungry. If the high-calorie food doesn't get into your house, it's not going to be on your dinner plate. That's a big win!

90. **TAKE A COFFEE-WALK BREAK.** Here's another one of my favorite suggestions for managing weight and burning more calories: always take a walk break every time you have a coffee/tea break. I have been doing this for years. Feel free to take the walk break after the coffee break or before. Depending on my mood at the moment, I always change up the sequence. Next, depending on my time, I will walk from 3 to 15 minutes. But I always walk briskly, because you burn more calories this way. When you walk at about 3 mph—a brisk pace—you burn 300% more calories than just sitting and sipping your coffee. An added benefit is that these coffee-walk breaks really positively contribute to your overall health.

91. **PUT YOUR FORK AND KNIFE DOWN BETWEEN BITES.** Definitely try this distinctive dining technique: put your fork and knife down between bites and chew your food slowly. A 2008 study in the *Journal of the Academy of Nutrition and Dietetics* showed that women ate on average 66 calories less by slowing their eating patterns. This technique can really contribute to successful weight loss over the long run. Remember, "Inch by inch, it's a cinch."

92. **EAT IN FRONT OF A MIRROR EVERY ONCE IN A WHILE.** Yes, I know this sounds really bizarre. However, a 2016 study in the *Journal of the Association for Consumer Research* found that when people watched themselves eat in a mirror they chose healthier options and ate fewer calories. The researchers explained that the presence of a mirror can make unhealthy food less tasty by increasing self-awareness.

93. **TAKE A WALK AFTER EACH MEAL.** Here's another favorite tip I share with all of my students: time permitting, take a brief 3 to 15 minute walk right after you eat a meal. The walk will help you burn some calories and it aids digestion. Researchers have found that a post-meal walk will also improve blood sugar levels. This is beneficial for keeping insulin from spiking and depositing fat.

94. **TAKE YOUR TIME GROCERY SHOPPING.** When you are shopping for food, you are moving about 2 miles/hour and burning 200% more calories than just sitting. That's a lot more calories than when you're just sitting and reading. As a result, I regularly encourage students to take their time grocery shopping and reap the benefits of this additional calorie burn. In fact, I encourage you to walk up and down *all* of the aisles before you go to the register. If you do this routine often and if you get into a habit of making your shopping last longer, you will be burning many more calories over the long run. Go for it!

95. **EAT WITH YOUR NONDOMINANT HAND.** This is a unique eating intervention, but it works. I know—it does seem to be awkward at first, but if you're prone to eating quickly, eating with your nondominant hand could help you slow down and chew your food slower. In the long run, you may actually eat less. How about giving it a few tries and then self-evaluating? It may be an option for you with some meals.

96. **GET ENOUGH SLEEP.** Studies show a lack of sleep has been linked with obesity. In fact, people who don't sleep well tend to weigh more than those who are regularly well rested. One reason is that people who sleep poorly are likely to be hungrier and consume more calories. If you're trying to cut calories and lose some weight, make sure you consistently get 7–9 hours of sleep each night.

97. **KEEP YOUR KITCHEN CLEAN.** When it feels like everything around you is chaotic and cluttered, keeping your diet under control becomes less of a priority. In a 2016 study published in *Environment and Behavior,* one hundred and one female college students participated in an experiment in which the difference between eating behavior in a clean, organized

kitchen and a messy, chaotic one was measured. The participants were given carrots, cookies, and crackers while they were in a kitchen and told to eat as much as they wanted. The participants in the messy, chaotic kitchen consumed more calories, mostly through cookies, than the participants in the clean, organized kitchen. The study shows that a less cluttered and less chaotic environment may lead people to snack less.

98. **ORDER FOOD BEFORE YOU'RE HUNGRY.** If your favorite lunch eatery has online ordering or a call-ahead option, take advantage of it. A 2016 study published in the *Journal of Marketing Research* found that people who selected catered food options at least an hour before eating tended to order fewer calories than people who ordered food at lunchtime and ate immediately. Waiting until you're hungry to decide what to eat increases your odds of overindulging, say the study researchers.

99. **GET A MASSAGE.** For many people, stress is a trigger for eating—and often more sugar, fat, and salt. Sometimes a simple shoulder and neck massage will release some of that built-up stress while helping you curb any stressful eating. You deserve it. Find a good friend, family member or companion with whom you can swap massages.

100. **GO AHEAD: IT'S OK TO GET A HEALTH COACH.** This is a worthy tip number 100. One way to improve any lifestyle behavior is by securing the services of a health coach. Health coaching, sometimes called wellness coaching, is an interactive form of coaching that promotes positive, sustainable behavioral change. An effective health coach encourages clients to listen to their inner wisdom, identify their values, and put their goals into action. Most health coaching interventions are delivered through telephone, web-based chatting, or a combination of face-to-face and web-based instruction. Your health practitioner may be able to personally refer you to some health coaching resources in your area, so start there. You can check the coach's credentials on the web. Studies show health coaching is quite effective at improving lifestyle behaviors that promote weight loss. Is this something you would consider?

MY SALUTATION TO YOU

THE WORLD HAS ADVANCED SO MUCH TECHNOLOGICALLY THAT WE NOW LIVE A LARGELY sedentary lifestyle. Many of us have sedentary jobs, do not do heavy work, watch sports as opposed to participating in them, take elevators and escalators, play computer games, text/talk for many minutes each day, and drive short distances instead of walking them. The chair has become our throne, resulting in a world where many people suffer from sitting diseases such as obesity, cardiovascular disease, and type 2 diabetes.

This may describe your own life, but that's not the end of this story. With the purchase of this book, you have taken the first step toward your physical activity journey—and to your new life. Having read the book and arrived at this point, I hope you feel empowered to take these major steps toward health and fitness, a journey that has no finish line but is endlessly rewarding, both physically and mentally. What you have learned over the course of this book—how HIIT training can get you into shape; winning ways to cut calories in your daily life; and numerous ideas for enhancing your health—will improve your life for years to come. (And very likely, extend it.)

Before I leave you, let's review the key takeaways from the book. Internalizing these messages above all else will help you succeed. Ready? Let's HIIT it one last time!

1. Make exercise a regular habit in your life.

2. Regardless of the diet you choose, find an eating lifestyle that allows you to best control your food intake. It's not the program that leads to success—it's your sincere efforts.

3.   Continued self-monitoring of your exercise and diet will always keep you on track.

4.   Always maintain a positive, problem-solving approach to stressors you face in life.

5.   Any negative disruptions in your life may lead to weight rebound.

6.   If you get off track with any of your fitness or dietary goals, first forgive yourself. Then determine what led you astray from your plan. Correct your trajectory and get back on the road to success.

7.   Always remind yourself of my philosophy: "Inch by inch, it's a cinch." The small steps approach is a formula for accomplishment that leads to great achievement outcomes, and most importantly, a healthier you!

8.   "For every 30, get your 3." For every 30 minutes of sitting, I want you to get at least 3 minutes of movement. Yes, more is better, but let's shoot for "For every 30, get your 3" as a start.

9.   On a daily basis, let healthy choices become your way of life.

10. Remind yourself regularly that you are on a lifelong journey. Enjoy living every moment to its fullest.

REFERENCES

SECTION 1: EXERCISE, HIIT, AND YOU!

CHAPTER 1: Exercise: The Quality of Life Super Pill

Booth, F. W., Roberts, C. K., and Laye, M. J. (2012). "Lack of exercise is a major cause of chronic diseases," *Comprehensive Physiology*, 2 (2), 1143-1211.

Dempsey, P. C., Larsen, R. N., Sethi, P., et al. (2016). "Benefits for type 2 diabetes of interrupting prolonged sitting with brief bouts of light walking or simple resistance activities," *Diabetes Care*, 39 (6), 964–972.

Diliberti, N., Bordi, P. L., Conklin, M. T., et al. (2004). "Increased portion size leads to increased energy intake in a restaurant meal," *Obesity*, 12 (3), 562-568.

Franklin, B. A. (2008). "Physical activity to combat chronic diseases and escalating health care costs: the unfilled prescription," *Current Sports Medicine Reports*, 7 (3), 122-125.

Kokkinos, P., Myers, J., Faselis, C., et al. (2010). "Exercise capacity and mortality in older men: a 20-year follow-up study," *Circulation*, 122 (8), 790-797.

MacAuley, D., Bauman, A., and Frémont, P. (2016). "Exercise: not a miracle cure, just good medicine," *British Journal of Sports Medicine*, 50 (18), 1107–1108.

Owen, N., Sparling, P. B., Healy, G. N., et al. (2010). "Sedentary behavior: emerging evidence for a new health risk," *Mayo Clinic Proceedings*, 85 (12), 1138-1141.

CHAPTER 2: What Is High-Intensity Interval Training (HIIT)?

Buchheit, M. and Laursen, P. B. (2013). "High-Intensity interval training, solutions to the programming puzzle: Part I: Cardiopulmonary Emphasis," *Sports Medicine*, 43 (5), 313-338.

Milanovic, Z., Sporis, G., and Weston, M. (2015). "Effectiveness of high-intensity interval training (HIT) and continuous endurance training for VO2max improvements: a systematic review and meta-analysis of controlled trials," *Sports Medicine*, 45 (10), 1469-1481.

Zhang, H., Tong, T. K., Qui, W., et al. (2017). "Comparable effects of high-intensity interval training and prolonged continuous exercise training on abdominal visceral fat reduction in obese young women," *Journal of Diabetes Research*, doi.org/10.1155/2017/5071740.

CHAPTER 3: What Are the Health Benefits of HIIT?

American Diabetic Association (2013). "Blood glucose and exercise." Retrieved from http://www.diabetes.org/food-and-fitness/fitness/get-started-safely/blood-glucose-control-and-exercise.html.

Blair, S. N., Kampert, J. B., Kohl, H. W., et al. (1996). "Influences of cardiorespiratory fitness and other precursors on cardiovascular disease and all-cause mortality in men and women," *Journal of the American Medical Association*, 276 (3), 205-210.

Boutcher, S. H. (2011). "High-intensity intermittent exercise and fat loss," *Journal of Obesity*, 2011, Article ID868305, doi: 10.1155/2011/868305.

Kessler, H. S., Sisson, S. B., and Short, K. R. (2012). "The potential for high-intensity interval training to reduce cardiometabolic disease risk," *Sports Medicine*, 42 (6), 489-509.

Knab, A. M., Shanely, R. A., Corbin, K. D., et al. (2011). "A 45-minute vigorous exercise bout increases metabolic rate for 14 hours," *Medicine & Science in Sports & Exercise*, 43 (9), 1643-1648.

Swain, D. P., and Franklin, B. A. (2006). "Comparison of cardioprotective benefits of vigorous versus moderate intensity aerobic exercise," *American Journal of Cardiology*, 97 (1), 141-147.

Talanian, J. L., Galloway, S. D. R., Heigenhauser, G. J. F., et al. (2007). "Two weeks of high-intensity aerobic interval training increases the capacity for fat oxidation during exercise in women," *Journal of Applied Physiology*, 102 (4), 1439-1447.

World Health Organization (2017) "Cardiovascular Diseases (CVDs)." Retrieved from http://www.who.int/mediacentre/factsheets/fs317/en/.

Zhang, H., Tong, T. K., Qui, W., et al. (2017). "Comparable effects of high-intensity interval training and prolonged continuous exercise training on abdominal visceral fat reduction in obese women," *Journal of Diabetes Research*, doi.org/10.1155/2017/5071740.

CHAPTER 4: How Does Your Body Power Your HIIT Workouts?

Kenney, W. L., Wilmore, J. H., and Costill, D. L. (2015). *Physiology of Sport and Exercise* (6th edition). Human Kinetics.

Kravitz, L. (2011). "Marvelous mitochondria!" *IDEA Fitness Journal*, 8 (5), 21-23.

Kravitz, L. (2005). "Lactate: Not guilty as charged," *IDEA Fitness Journal*, 2 (6), 23-25.

CHAPTER 5: Ten Steps to Succeed in an Exercise Program

Bravata, D. M., Smith-Spangler, C., Sundaram, V., et al. (2007). "Using pedometers to increase physical activity and improve health," *Journal of the American Medical Association*, 298 (19), 2296-2304.

Koeneman, M. A., Verheijden, M. W., Chinapaw, M. J. M., et al. (2011). "Determinants of physical activity and exercise in healthy older adults: a systematic review," *International Journal of Behavioral Nutrition and Physical Activity*, 8, 142, doi: 10.1186/1479-5868-8-142.

CHAPTER 6: Do It Right: Avoid These Exercise Mistakes

Kravitz, L. (2016). *Anybody's Guide to Total Fitness* (11th edition), Kendall Hunt Publishing Company, Dubuque, IA.

CHAPTER 7: Time for Your Heart Health Pre-Check

Benjamin, E. J., Blaha, M. J., Chiuve, S. E., et al. (2017). "Heart disease and stroke statistics—2017 update: a report from the American Heart Association," *Circulation*, 135 (10), e146-e603.

Levine, H. (2017). "The healing power of a heart-healthy diet," *Consumer Reports*, 82 (5), 32.

Pescatello, L. S., Arena, R., Riebe, D., et al. (2014). *ACSM's Guidelines for Exercise Testing and Prescription* (9th edition). Philadelphia: Wolters Kluwer/Lippincott Williams & Wilkins.

Whelton, P. K., Carey, R. M., Aronow, W. S., et al. (2017). "2017 ACC/AHA/AAPA/ABC/ACPM/AGS/APhA/ASH/ASPC/NMA/PCNA Guideline for the Prevention, Detection, Evaluation, and Management of High Blood Pressure in Adults," *Journal of the American College of Cardiology*, May 2018, 71 (19) e127-e248.

CHAPTER 8: Let's Get Up and Start Moving Now!

Colberg, S. R., Sigal, R. J., Yardley, J. E., et al. (2016). "Physical activity/exercise and diabetes: a position statement of the American Diabetes Association," *Diabetes Care*, 39 (11), 2065-2079.

Dempsey, P. C., Larsen, R. N., Sethi, P., et al. (2016). "Benefits for type 2 diabetes of interrupting prolonged sitting with brief bouts of light walking or simple resistance activities," *Diabetes Care*, 39 (6), 964-972.

Hamilton, M. T., Healy, G. N., Dunstan, D. W., et al. (2008). "Too little exercise and too much sitting: inactivity physiology and the need for new recommendations on sedentary behavior," *Current Cardiovascular Risk Reports*, 2, 292-298.

Katzmarzyk, P. T., Church, T. S., Craig, C. L., et al. (2009). "Sitting time and mortality from all causes, cardiovascular disease, and cancer," *Medicine & Science in Sports & Exercise*, 41 (5), 998-1005.

Morris, J. N., and Crawford, M. D. (1958). "Coronary heart disease and physical activity of work," *British Medical Journal*, 2 (5111), 1485–1496.

Owen, N., Bauman, A., and Brown, W. (2009). "Too much sitting: a novel and important predictor of chronic disease risk?" *British Journal of Sports Medicine*, 43 (2), 81-83.

Pescatello, L. S., Arena, R., Riebe, D., et al. (2014). *ACSM's Guidelines for Exercise Testing and Prescription* (9th edition). Philadelphia: Wolters Kluwer/Lippincott Williams & Wilkins.

SECTION 2: OPTIMAL WEIGHT (FAT) LOSS STRATEGIES THAT WORK!

CHAPTER 9: Successful Weight Management; "Inch by Inch, It's a Cinch"

Centers for Disease Control and Prevention (2018). "Adult obesity facts." Retrieved from https://www.cdc.gov/obesity/data/adult.html.

Fabricatore, A. N., and Wadden, T. A. (2003). "Treatment of obesity. An Overview," *Clinical Diabetes*, 21 (2), 6–72.

Hall, K. D., Heymsfield, S. B., Kemnitz, J. W., et al. (2012). "Energy balance and its components: implications for body weight regulation," *American Journal of Clinical Nutrition*, 95(4), 989-994.

Hill, J. O. (2009). "Can a small-changes approach help address the obesity epidemic? A report of the Joint Task Force on the American Society for Nutrition, Institute of Food Technologists, and International Food Information Council," *American Journal of Clinical Nutrition*, 89 (2), 477-484.

Sifferlin, A. (2017). "This diet may help you lose weight," *Time*, June 5, 50-55.

World Health Organization (2017). "Obesity and Overweight." Retrieved from http://www.who.int/en/news-room/fact-sheets/detail/obesity-and-overweight.

CHAPTER 10: Lessons from *The Biggest Loser*

Albuquerque, D., Stice, D., Rodriguez-Lopez. R., et al. (2015). "Current review of genetics of human obesity: from molecular mechanisms to an evolutionary perspective," *Molecular Genetics and Genomics*, 290 (4), 1191–1221.

Fothergill, E., Guo, J., Howard, L., et al. (2016). "Persistent metabolic adaptation 6 years after 'The Biggest Loser' competition," *Obesity*, 24 (8), 1612–1619.

Pietilainen, K. H., Saarni, S. E., Kaprio, J., et al. (2012). "Does dieting make you fat? A twin study," *International Journal of Obesity*, 36, 456–464.

Sumithran, P., Pendegast, L. A., Delbridge, E., et al. (2011). "Long-term persistence of hormonal adaptations to weight loss," *New England Journal of Medicine*, 365, 1597-1604.

Wang, Z., Heshka, S., Gallagher, D., et al. (2000). "Resting energy expenditure-fat-free mass relationship: new insights provided by body composition modeling," *American Journal of Physiology-Endocrinology and Metabolism*, 279 (3), E539–E545.

CHAPTER 11: Secrets from Real-Life Biggest Losers

McGuire, M. T., Wing, R. R., Klem, M. L., et al. (1999). "What predicts weight regain in a group of successful weight losers?" *Journal of Consulting and Clinical Psychology*, 67 (2), 177-185.

NWCR. (2017). "NWCR Facts." National Weight Control Registry. Retrieved from http://www.nwcr.ws.

Wing, R. R., and Phelan, S. (2005). "Long-term weight loss maintenance," *American Journal of Clinical Nutrition*, 82 (1), 222S-225S.

CHAPTER 12: What's the Healthiest Diet for Me?

Chung, H. Y., Cesari, M., Anton, S., et al. (2010). "Molecular inflammation: underpinnings of aging and age-related diseases," *Ageing Research Review*, 8 (1), 18–30.

Crous-Bou, M., Fung, T. T., Prescott, J., et al. (2014). "Mediterranean diet and telomere length in Nurses' Health Study: population based cohort study," *British Medical Journal* doi: 10.1136/bmj.g6674.

Krauss, J., Farzaneh-Far, R., Puterman, E., et al. (2011). "Physical fitness and telomere length in patients with coronary heart disease: findings from the Heart and Soul Study," PLOS ONE, 6 (11), e26983. doi:10.1371/journal.pone.0026983.

Rader, D. J. (2017). "Mediterranean approach to improving high-density lipoprotein function," *Circulation*, 135, 644–647.

CHAPTER 13: Low-Carbohydrate versus Low-Fat Diets: What Is the Verdict?

Colberg, S. R., Sigal, R. J., Yardley, J. E., et al. (2016). "Physical activity/exercise and diabetes: a position statement of the American Diabetes Association," *Diabetes Care*, 39 (11), 2065-2079.

Hall, K. D., Bernis, T., Brychta, R., et al. (2015). "Calorie for calorie, dietary fat restriction results in more body fat loss than carbohydrate restriction in people with obesity," *Cell Metabolism*, 22 (3), 427–436.

Hall, K. D., Chen, K. Y., Guo, J., et al. (2016). "Energy expenditure and body composition changes after an isocaloric ketogenic diet in overweight and obese men," *American Journal of Clinical Nutrition*, 104 (2), 324–333.

Jensen, M. D., Ryan, D. H., Apovian, C. M., et al. (2014). "2013 AHA/ACC/TOS Guideline for the management of overweight and obesity in adults," *Circulation*. 2014;129 [25 Suppl 2], S102-S138.

Shai, I., Schwarzfuchs, D., Henkin, Y., et al. (2008) "Weight loss with a low-carbohydrate, Mediterranean, or low-fat diet," *New England Journal of Medicine*, 359, 229–241.

CHAPTER 14: The Stress-Cortisol-Obesity Connection

Bjorntorp, P. (2001). "Do stress reactions cause abdominal obesity and comorbidities?" *Obesity Reviews*, 2 (2), 73–86.

Montes, M. V., and Kravitz, L. (2011). "Unraveling the stress-eating-obesity knot," *IDEA Fitness Journal*, 8 (2), 45–50.

NIH. (2001). "ATP III At-A-Glance: Quick Desk Reference." Retrieved from https://www.nhlbi.nih.gov/files/docs/guidelines/atglance.pdf.

Pasquali, R. (2012). "The hypothalamic-pituitary-adrenal axis and sex hormones in chronic stress and obesity: pathophysiological and clinical aspects," *Annals of the New York Academy of Sciences*, 1264 (1), 20–35.

Attie, A. D., and Scherer, P. E. (2009). "Adipocyte metabolism and obesity," *Journal of Lipid Research,* 50, S395-S399.

Bacon, L., Stern, J. S., Van Loan, M. D., et al. (2005). "Size acceptance and intuitive eating improve health for obese, female chronic dieters," *Journal of the American Diet Association,* 105 (6), 929–936.

Bangalore, S., Fayyad, R., Laskey, R., et al. (2017), "Body-weight fluctuations and outcomes in coronary disease," *New England Journal of Medicine,* 376, 1332-1340.

Bao, Y., Han, J., and Hu, F. B. (2013). "Association of nut consumption with total and cause-specific mortality," *New England Journal of Medicine,* 369, 2001-2011.

Berkeley Wellness. (2017). "Nutrition Bars: Do They Deliver?" University of California, *Berkeley Wellness Letter,* May 4.

Berkeley Wellness. (2017). "13 heart-healthy steps for women (and men, too)," University of California, *Berkeley Wellness Letter,* May 5.

Calton, J. B. (2010). "Prevalence of micronutrient deficiency in popular diet plans," *Journal of the International Society of Sports Nutrition,* http://doi.org/10.1186/1550-2783-7-24.

Celiac Disease Foundation, (2017). "What is celiac disease?" Retrieved from https://celiac.org/celiac-disease/understanding-celiac-disease-2/what-is-celiac-disease/.

Després, J. P. (2015). "Obesity and cardiovascular disease: weight loss is not the only target," *Canadian Journal of Cardiology,* 31 (2), 216-222.

Healthy Lifestyle (2017). "Caffeine: how much is too much?" Mayo Clinic. Retrieved from http://www.mayoclinic.org/healthy-lifestyle/nutrition-and-healthy-eating/in-depth/caffeine/art-20045678.

Hurley, J., and Liebman, B. (2015). "Not milk?" *Nutrition Action Healthletter,* 42 (1), 13–15.

Jeukendrup, A. E., and Randell, R. (2011). "Fat burners: nutrition supplements that increase fat metabolism," *Obesity Reviews,* 12 (10), 841–851.

Knize, M. G., and Felton, J. S. (2005). "Formation and human risk of carcinogenic heterocyclic amines formed from natural precursors in meat," *Nutrition Reviews,* 63 (5), 158–165.

Kravitz, L. (2016). *Anybody's Guide to Total Fitness* (11th edition). Kendall Hunt Publishing Company, Dubuque, IA.

Kyro, C., and Tjonneland, A. (2016). "Whole grains and public health," *BMJ,* 2016, 353:i3046.

Liebman, B. (2015). "Are multivitamins a waste of money?" NutritionAction.com. Retrieved from https://www.nutritionaction.com/daily/dietary-supplements/are-multivitamins-a-waste-of-money/.

Liebman, B. (2015). "Bye bye beef?" *Nutrition Action Healthletter*, 42 (8), 3–7.

Liebman, B. (2017). "What makes us eat too much," *Nutrition Action Healthletter*, 44 (3), 3–6.

Miller, J. L. (2013). "Iron deficiency anemia: a common and curable disease," *Cold Spring Harbor Perspectives in Medicine*, doi: 10.1101/cshperspect.a011866.

Ness-Abramof, R., and Apovian, C. M. (2008). "Waist circumference measurement in clinical practice," *Nutrition in Clinical Practice*, 23 (4), 397–404.

NIH, National Cancer Institute. Retrieved from https://www.cancer.gov.

Paoli, A., Marcolin, G., Zonin, F., et al. (2011). "Exercising fasting or fed to enhance fat loss? Influence of food intake on respiratory ratio and excess postexercise oxygen consumption after a bout of endurance training," *International Journal of Sport Nutrition and Exercise Metabolism*, 21 (1), 48-54.

Romieu, I., Dossus, L, Barquera, S., et al. (2017). "Energy balance and obesity: what are the main drivers?" *Cancer Causes & Control*, 28 (3), 247–258.

Thom, E., Wadstein, J., and Gudmundsen, O. (2001). "Conjugated linoleic acid reduces body fat in healthy exercising humans," *Journal of International Medical Research*, 29 (5), 392–396.

Trepanowski, J. F., Kroeger, C. M., Barnosky, A., et al. (2017). "Effect of alternate-day fasting on weight loss, weight maintenance, and cardioprotection among metabolically healthy obese adults: a randomized clinical trial," *JAMA Internal Medicine*, 177 (7), 930–938.

US Department of Health and Human Services and U.S. Department of Agriculture. 2015–2020 *Dietary Guidelines for Americans* (8th edition). December 2015. Retrieved from http://health.gov/dietaryguidelines/2015/.

Weaver, A. M., and Kravitz, L. (2014). "Understanding iron-deficiency anemia & sports anemia," *IDEA Fitness Journal*, 11 (8), 16–19.

World Health Organization. "Body Mass Index-BMI." Retrieved from http://www.euro.who.int/en/health-topics/disease-prevention/nutrition/a-healthy-lifestyle/body-mass-index-bmi.

Zeratsky, K. (2015). "Which spread is better for my heart—butter or margarine?" Mayo Clinic. Retrieved from http://www.mayoclinic.org/healthy-lifestyle/nutrition-and-healthy-eating/expert-answers/butter-vs-margarine/faq-20058152.

SECTION 3: LET'S HIIT THE WORKOUTS!

CHAPTER 16: Pre-Exercise Fundamentals

Kravitz, L. (2016). *Anybody's Guide to Total Fitness* (11th edition). Kendall Hunt Publishing Company, Dubuque, IA.

CHAPTER 17: Why Your Workout Warm-Up and Cooldown Are so Important

Kravitz, L. (2016). *Anybody's Guide to Total Fitness* (11th edition). Kendall Hunt Publishing Company, Dubuque, IA.

CHAPTER 18: How Hard Should I Exercise?

Borg, G. A. V. (1982). "Psychological bases of perceived exertion," *Medicine & Science in Sports & Exercise*, 14 (5), 377-381.

Persinger, R., Foster, C., Gibson, M., et al. (2004). "Consistency of the talk test for exercise prescription," *Medicine & Science Sports & Exercise*, 36 (9), 1632-1636.

CHAPTER 19: Your HIIT Workouts Plan

Garber, C. E., Blissmer, B., Deschenes, M. R., et al. (2011) "American College of Sports Medicine position stand. Quantity and quality of exercise for developing and maintaining cardiorespiratory, musculoskeletal, and neuromotor fitness in apparently healthy adults: guidance for prescribing exercise," *Medicine & Science in Sports & Exercise*, 43 (7),1334-1359.

Zhang, H., Tong, T. K., Qui, W., et al. (2017). "Comparable effects of high-intensity interval training and prolonged continuous exercise training on abdominal visceral fat reduction in obese women," *Journal of Diabetes Research*, doi.org/10.1155/2017/5071740.

CHAPTER 20: Your HIIT Workouts—Enjoy!

Akers, A., Barton, J., Cossey, R., et al. (2012). "Visual color perception in green exercise: positive effects on mood and perceived exertion," *Environmental Science & Technology*, 46 (16), 8661-8666.

Burgomaster, K. A., Howarth, K. R., Phillips, S. M., et al. (2008). "Similar metabolic adaptations during exercise after low volume sprint interval and traditional endurance training in humans," *Journal of Applied Physiology*, 586 (1), 151–160.

Borg, G. A. V. (1982). "Psychological bases of perceived exertion," *Medicine & Science in Sports & Exercise*, 14 (5), 377–381.

Gibala, M. J. (2015). "Physiological adaptations to low-volume high-intensity interval training," *Sports Science Exchange*, 28 (139), 1–6.

Gosselin, L. E., Kozlowski, K. F., DeVinney-Boymel, L., et al. (2012) "Metabolic response of different high-intensity aerobic interval exercise protocols," *Journal of Strength and Conditioning Research*, 26 (10), 2866–2871.

Helgerud, J. K, Hoydal, K., Wang, E. (2007). "Aerobic high-intensity intervals improve VO2max more than moderate training," *Medicine & Science in Sports & Exercise*, 39 (4), 665–671.

Kravitz, L. (2016). *Anybody's Guide to Total Fitness* (11th edition). Kendall Hunt Publishing Company, Dubuque, IA.

Moriarty, T. M., Escobar, K., Nunez, T., et al. (2017). "The physiology of spring interval training," *IDEA Fitness Journal*," 14 (4), 40–49.

Smith, T. P., Coombes, J. S., and Geraghty, D. P. (2003). "Optimising high-intensity treadmill training using the running speed at maximal O(2) uptake and the time for which this can be maintained," *European Journal of Applied Physiology*, 89 (34), 337–343.

Trapp, E. G., Chisholm, D. J., Freund, J., and Boutcher, S. H. (2008). "The effects of high-intensity intermittent exercise training on fat loss and fasting insulin levels of young women," *International Journal of Obesity*, 32, 684–691.

CHAPTER 21: The Future of HIIT Workouts—25 MORE Workouts!

Kravitz, L. (2016*). Anybody's Guide to Total Fitness* (11th edition). Kendall Hunt Publishing Company, Dubuque, IA.

Pescatello, L. S., Arena, R., Riebe, D., et al. (2014). *ACSM's Guidelines for Exercise Testing and Prescription* (9th edition). Philadelphia: Wolters Kluwer/Lippincott Williams & Wilkins.

Skidmore, B. L., Jones, M. T., Blegen, M., et al. (2012). "Acute effects of three different circuit weight training protocols on blood lactate, heart rate, and rating of perceived exertion in recreationally active women," *Journal of Sports Science and Medicine*, 11 (4), 660–668.

SECTION 4: 100 WINNING WAYS TO CUT CALORIES IN YOUR DAILY LIFE

Andrade, A. M., Greene, G. W., and Melanson, K. J. (2008). "Eating slowly led to decreases in energy intake within meals in healthy women," *Journal of the Academy of Nutrition and Dietetics*, 108 (7), 1186–1191.

Benton, D. (2015). "Portion size: what we know and what we need to know," *Critical Reviews in Food Science and Nutrition*, 55 (7), 988-1004.

Bray, G. A., and Popkin, B. M. (2014). "Dietary sugar and body weight: have we reached a crisis in the epidemic of obesity and diabetes?" *Diabetes Care*, 37 (4), 950-956.

Centers for Disease Control and Prevention (2015). "Rethink your drink." Retrieved from https://www.cdc.gov/healthyweight/healthy_eating/drinks.html.

Cheskin, L., Davis, L. J., Lipsky, L. M. (2008). "Lack of energy compensation over 4 days when white button mushrooms are substituted for beef," *Appetite*, 51 (1), 50-57.

Colberg, S. R., Zarrabi, L., Bennington, L., et al. (2009). "Postprandial walking is better for lowering the glycemic effect of dinner than pre-dinner exercise in type 2 diabetic individuals," *Journal of the American Medical Directors Association*, 10 (6), 394-397.

Consumer Reports (2015). "Why eating the right breakfast is so important." Retrieved from http://www.consumerreports.org/cro/magazine/2014/10/why-eating-the-right-breakfast-is-so-important/index.html.

Coughlin, J. W., and Smith, M. T. (2014). "Sleep, obesity, and weight loss in adults: is there a rationale for providing sleep interventions in the treatment of obesity?" *International Review of Psychiatry*, 26 (2), 177–188.

Daniels, M. C., and Popkin, B. M. (2010). "Impact of water intake on energy intake and weight status: a systematic review," *Nutrition Reviews*, 68 (9), 505–521.

Davy, B. M., Dennis, E. A., Dengo, A. L., et al., (2008). "Water consumption reduces energy intake at a breakfast meal in obese older adults," *Journal of the Academy of Nutrition and Dietetics*, 108 (7), 1236–1239.

Diliberti, N., Bordi, P. L., Conklin, M. T., et al. (2004). "Increased portion size leads to increased energy intake in a restaurant meal," *Obesity*, 12 (3), 562-568.

Doubnerova, V. (2013) "Is drinking of coffee and using of cardamom in the kitchen beneficial for our health?" *Biochemistry & Analytical Biochemistry*, 2:e134. Doi:10.4172/2161-1009.1000e134.

Flood, J. E., and Rolls, B. J. (2007). "Soup preloads in a variety of forms reduce meal energy intake," *Appetite*, 49 (3), 626-634.

Gardner, A. (2015). "High fiber diets and weight loss," WebMD. Retrieved from https://www.webmd.com/diet/features/fiber-weight-control#1.

Gurevich, P. (2014). "How many calories does dabbing the grease off a pizza slice save you?" *Labdoor*. Retrieved from https://labdoor.com/article/how-many-calories-does-dabbing-the-grease-off-a-pizza-slice-save-you.

Himaya, A., and Louis-Sylvestre, J. (1998). "The effect of soup on satiation," *Appetite*, 30 (2), 199-210.

Hoffmann, J. C., Mittal, S., Hoffman, C. H., et al. (2016). "Combating the health risks of sedentary behavior in the contemporary radiology reading room," *American Journal of Roentgenology*, 206 (6), 1135–1140.

Houchins, J. A., Tan, S. Y., Campbell, W. W., et al. (2012). "Effects of fruit and vegetable, consumed in solid vs beverage forms, on acute and chronic appetitive responses in lean and obese adults," *International Journal of Obesity*, 37, 1109–1115.

Hu, F. B. (2013). "Resolved: there is sufficient scientific evidence that decreasing sugar-sweetened beverage consumption will reduce the prevalence of obesity and obesity-related diseases," *Obesity Reviews*, 14 (8), 606–619.

Jami, A. (2016). "Healthy reflections: the influence of mirror-induced self-awareness on taste perceptions," *Journal of the Association for Consumer Research*, 1 (1), 57–70.

Kruger, J., Blanck, H. M., and Gillespie, C. (2008). "Dietary practices, dining out behavior, and physical activity correlates of weight loss maintenance," *Preventing Chronic Disease*, 5 (1), A11.

Leidy, H. J., Clifton, P. M., Astrup, A., et al. (2015). "The role of protein in weight loss and maintenance," *American Journal of Clinical Nutrition*, 101 (6), 1320S–1329S.

Levine, J. A., Schleusner, S. J., and Jensen, M. D. (2000). "Energy expenditure of nonexercise activity," *American Journal of Clinical Nutrition*, 72 (6), 1451–1454.

Ma, Y., Bertone, E. R., Stanek III, E. J. (2003). "Association between eating patterns and obesity in a free-living US adult population," *American Journal of Epidemiology*, 158 (1), 85–92.

Macht, M. (1999). "Characteristics of eating in anger, fear, sadness and joy," *Appetite*, 33 (2), 129–139.

Mantzios, M., and Wilson, J. C. (2015). "Mindfulness, eating behaviors, and obesity: a review and reflection on current findings," *Current Obesity Reports*, 4 (1), 141–146.

McClain, A. D., van den Bos, W., Matheson, D., et al. (2013). "Visual illusions and plate design: the effects of plate rim widths and rim coloring on perceived food portion size," *International Journal of Obesity*, 38, 657–662.

Moore, L. V., and Thompson, F. E. (2015). "Adults meeting fruit and vegetable intake recommendations-United States, 2013," *MMWR Morbidity and Mortality Weekly Report*, 64 (26), 709–713.

Oldham-Cooper, R. E., Hardman, C. A., Nicoll, C. E., et al. (2011). "Playing a computer game during lunch affects fullness, memory for lunch, and later snack intake," *American Journal of Clinical Nutrition*, 93 (2), 308–313.

Parretti, H. M., Aveyard, P., Blannin, A., et al. (2015). "Efficacy of water preloading before main meals as a strategy for weight loss in primary care patients with obesity: RCT," *Obesity*, 23 (9), 1785–1791.

Robinson, E., Aveyard, P., Daley, A., et al. (2013). "Eating attentively: a systematic review and meta-analysis of the effect of food intake memory and awareness on eating," *American Journal of Clinical Nutrition*, 97 (4), 728–742.

Robinson, E., Kersbergen, I., and Higgs, S. (2014). "Eating 'attentively' reduces later energy consumption in overweight and obese females," *British Journal of Nutrition*, 112 (4), 657661.

Rolls, B. J., Roe, L. S., and Meengs, J. S. (2010). "Portion size can be used strategically to increase vegetable consumption in adults," *American Journal of Clinical Nutrition*, 91 (4), 913–922.

Shah, M., Copeland, J., Dart, L., et al. (2014). "Slower eating speed lowers energy intake in normal-weight but not overweight/obese subjects," *Journal of the Academy of Nutrition and Dietetics*, 114 (3), 393–402.

Shearrer, G. E., O'Reilly, G. A., Belcher, B. R., et al. (2016). "The impact of sugar sweetened beverage intake on hunger and satiety in minority adolescents," *Appetite*, 97, 43–48.

Shechter, A., Grandner, M. A., and St-Onge, M. P. (2014). "The role of sleep in the control of food intake," *American Journal of Lifestyle Medicine*, 8 (6), 371–374.

Taheri, S., Lin, L., Austin, D., et al. (2004). "Short sleep duration is associated with reduced leptin, elevated ghrelin, and increased body mass index," *PLOS Medicine*, 1 (3), e62.

Urban, L. E., Weber, J. L., Heyman, M. B., et al. (2016). "Energy contents of frequently ordered restaurant meals and comparison with human energy requirements and US Department of Agriculture Database Information: a multisite randomized study," *Journal of the Academy of Nutrition and Dietetics*, 116 (4), 590–598.

VanEpps, E. M., Downs, J. S., and Loewenstein, G. (2016). "Advance ordering for healthier eating? Field experiments on the relationship between the meal order–consumption time delay and meal content," *Journal of Marketing Research*, 53 (3), 369–380.

Vartanian, L. R., Kernan, K. M., Wansink, B. (2016). "Clutter, chaos, and overconsumption: the role of mind-set in stressful and chaotic food environments," *Environment and Behavior*, 49 (2), 215–223.

Wansink, B., Van Ittersum, K., and Painter, J. E. (2006). "Ice cream illusions: bowls, spoons, and self-served portion sizes," *American Journal of Preventive Medicine*, 31 (3), 240–243.

Wansink, B., and Cheney, M. M. (2005). "Super bowls: serving bowl size and food consumption," *JAMA, 293* (14), 1723–1728.

Wansink, B., and Van Ittersum, K. (2013). "Portion size me: plate-size induced consumption norms and win-win solutions for reducing food intake and waste," *Journal of Experimental Psychology: Applied,* 19 (4), 320–332.

Wolfson, J. A., and Bleich, S. N. (2015). "Is cooking at home associated with better diet quality or weight-loss intention?" *Public Health Nutrition,* 18 (8), 1397–1406.

ACKNOWLEDGMENTS

I WISH TO THANK MY GREAT PHOTOGRAPHER, JACOB COVELL, AND MY FABULOUS EXERCISE models, Anna M. Welch, Kelsey Bourbeau, Mary Guiterrez, Roberto A. Nava, Terence Moriarty, and Torry Amelio. A special credit to Terence Moriarty for working with me on some cutting-edge research. To Justine Dineen, thank you for always being so thoughtful and supportive of me on my many projects. I am most grateful to my incredible editor, Adam Rosen. Adam, you have a wonderful way of making writing come alive. It is with great enthusiasm and admiration that I acknowledge, applaud, and thank my publisher and director of editorial, Julia Abramoff. Julia, you are marvelous at your craft. And lastly, I recognize and salute my students who provide me with the motivation and inspiration to always strive to achieve my best.

ABOUT THE AUTHOR

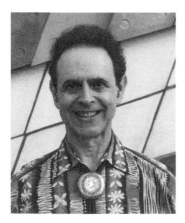

DR. LEN KRAVITZ HAS THIRTY-SIX YEARS OF EXPERIENCE AS a researcher, writer, and speaker on exercise science and fitness education. He is the coordinator of the Exercise Science program at the University of New Mexico and an associate professor in its Department of Health, Exercise and Sports Sciences, a position that earned him an Outstanding Teacher of the Year award. Dr. Kravitz has a master's degree in physical education and a PhD with an emphasis in exercise science and health promotion. He is the author of *Anybody's Guide to Total Fitness*, now in its eleventh edition with nearly one hundred thousand copies sold, and *Essentials of Eccentric Training*, and has published more than three hundred peer-reviewed articles in health and fitness publications. Dr. Kravitz regularly travels as a speaker on physical fitness and has presented at more than one thousand fitness and exercise science conferences around the world. He is the recipient of a wide variety of honors in the fitness industry, including an induction into the National Fitness Hall of Fame. Dr. Kravitz lives in Albuquerque, New Mexico.

PHYSICAL ACTIVITY TRACKER

Aim for two HIIT training workouts a week, with any other aerobic workouts being steady-state workouts (such as brisk walking, cycling, or swimming). When ready for more of a challenge, increase your workout frequency to a third HIIT workout a week. Spread your HIIT workouts throughout the week. Track all of your workouts with this physical activity tracker.

DATE	WORKOUT YOU DID	DURATION	COMMENTS ON WORKOUT

DATE	WORKOUT YOU DID	DURATION	COMMENTS ON WORKOUT

DATE	WORKOUT YOU DID	DURATION	COMMENTS ON WORKOUT

HIIT Your Limit

DATE	WORKOUT YOU DID	DURATION	COMMENTS ON WORKOUT

DATE	WORKOUT YOU DID	DURATION	COMMENTS ON WORKOUT